T0091788

Dealing with Child Abuse and Neglect as Public Health Problems

Jack C. Westman

Dealing with Child Abuse and Neglect as Public Health Problems

Prevention and the Role of Juvenile Ageism

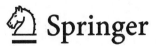 Springer

Jack C. Westman
School of Medicine and Public Health
University of Wisconsin–Madison
Madison, WI, USA

ISBN 978-3-030-05896-8   ISBN 978-3-030-05897-5   (eBook)
https://doi.org/10.1007/978-3-030-05897-5

Library of Congress Control Number: 2018966341

This Springer imprint is published by the registered company Springer Nature Switzerland AG
The registered company address is: Gewerbestrasse 11, 6330 Cham, Switzerland

Acknowledgments

Without the experience of raising three sons with my wife, ongoing affection and respect for three daughters-in-law, and participating in the lives of nine grandchildren, I would not know firsthand all of the rewards and the vicissitudes of parenthood.

In addition, my work with systems that affect children and families over five decades brought me together with professionals from a variety of disciplines in Wisconsin Cares, Inc., an advocacy organization for families. I am especially indebted to Norma Berkowitz, Paul Brandl, Glen Cain, Tom Corbett, Jack DeWitt, Ethel Dunn, Martin Fliegel, Vern Haubrich, Jim Hickman, Margo Melli, Frank Newgent, Dave Nordstrom, Gary Ranum, Tom Schleitwiler, Florian Smoczynski, Bernie Stumbras, Bob Sundby, Jan Van Vleck, and Sherwood Zink. Through Wisconsin Cares, Inc., we stimulated awareness of how struggling families affect their members, their communities, and society as well as how to strengthen these families, many of which began with adolescent parents. I greatly appreciate the suggestions and editing provided by Denis Donovan.

I am most grateful to the children, teenagers, and adults who have permitted me to share their lives in clinical and organizational settings.

Although this book is based upon cited scientific research, I have written it in an informal style for the convenience of a general audience.

Contents

List of Figures

List of Tables

Chapter 1
Introduction

The Gross Domestic Product measures everything except that which makes life worthwhile.

Robert F. Kennedy

University of Kansas, March 18, 1968 (Kennedy 1968)

A baby's smile warms our hearts and draws us in. We human beings are hardwired to care for newborn babies to ensure the survival of our species. Yet more than 11 million children in the United States have been born to parents who damaged them by serious neglect and/or abuse. Their fate is determined by the Cradle to Prison/Welfare Dependency Pipeline so well outlined by the Children's Defense Fund (2007).

Why do we permit babies to have three strikes against them at birth and endanger our nation's future? The most obvious reason is that we act as if we do not know that parents have the power to enhance or detract from our nation's prosperity. We leave the future of our children with parents who neglect and/or abuse them to separate professions and social services that try to help these struggling families but cannot deal with the obvious causes of intergenerational poverty, crime, and welfare dependency. Moreover, these unconnected, crisis-recoil responses to problems cannot apply what we know really works to prevent them in the first place and to help families in crises. If this fragmented approach was applied to health care, we would immunize only a fraction of our population and then treat only a fraction of the individuals who became infected. The result would be pandemics of diseases as we now see with the educational failures, endemic crime, welfare dependency, drug addiction, and intergenerational poverty that result from child abuse and neglect.

We no longer can afford to ignore the causes of our social problems. United Nations statistician Howard Friedman carefully documented the declining international status of the United States in his book *The Measure of a Nation* (Friedman 2012). He based this on the following facts as a basis for comparing America with other developed nations:

© Springer Nature Switzerland AG 2019
J. C. Westman, *Dealing with Child Abuse and Neglect as Public Health Problems*, https://doi.org/10.1007/978-3-030-05897-5_1

- Americans have the lowest life expectancy.
- Americans are at least two times more likely to be murdered and four times more likely to be incarcerated.
- America shows the greatest disparity between the rich and the poor.
- The United States signed the United Nations *Convention on the Rights of the Child*, but it is the only United Nations member that has not ratified it.

While America focuses on current unemployment, the national debt, and terrorism, the ailments that infect it are being ignored. Especially dangerous is the decline in thriving families that threatens the prosperity and security of our nation. This decline in family well-being deprives us of parents who are able to develop the characters and competencies of our young citizens…America's greatest natural resource.

This book is the story of my gradual recognition as a psychiatrist and volunteer lobbyist with state and federal governments that we live in a juvenile ageist society. Americans readily deplore prejudice based on age against the elderly who can vote, while we ignore prejudice based on age against our even more helpless children who cannot vote. We deprive millions of young people of opportunities to become productive citizens as we say we are devoted to them. We can overcome this hidden prejudice and resulting discrimination by first accepting its existence and then by ensuring that all newborn babies have competent parents who can give them an opportunity to succeed in life.

The vast majority of struggling families still do not receive the help they need. Fortunately, the coordinated interdisciplinary approach I developed in the 1970s is now being applied in most communities throughout our nation in the form of Wraparound Teams. When mental health, social services, educational, law enforcement, and court professionals work together with a family as a team—like the health-care system is set up to do—even the most difficult family problems can be resolved.

Most importantly, with a few notable exceptions like James Heckman and Hazel Henderson, economists have not considered the role parenthood plays in our nation's economy. Competent parents who raise a child to become a productive citizen contribute $1.4 million to our economy in earnings and taxes during that child's adulthood. Incompetent parents who abuse and neglect their children cost our economy $2.8 million for each child in lost earnings and taxes and in the costs of special education, crime, and welfare dependency (see Appendices 1 and 2). As a result, an estimated 23% of our state and 45% of our county expenditures are related to struggling families.

Fully one-third of our children and adolescents are not doing well. Over 11 million have been seriously damaged by neglect and/or abuse. School failures, addictions, crime, and welfare dependency are largely preventable if we simply would do one thing: ensure that all newborn babies have competent parents. My central theme is a fact that unfortunately is not reflected in popular beliefs:

> The unpaid career of parenthood is more important for the health of our nation's economy than paid jobs.

This theme is based on the following indisputable facts:

1. Without parenthood, we will not have citizens.
2. Without competent parents, we will not have competent citizens and workers.
3. Without competent citizens and workers, our economy will not prosper.

Incredibly, we presume that anyone who conceives a child is capable of raising that child. We do little to prepare individuals for the most important role in our society. We have no standards or guidelines for parenthood except for people who want to adopt children...and pets! We equate the human right to procreate with parental rights. Moreover, our society's emphasis on materialism and individualism distracts parents from forming and sustaining the attachment bonds that are the very foundation of every child's emotional, cognitive, social, and moral development.

American society clings to the illusion that we treasure our children and support parents...especially by adulating parents who sacrifice in order to give their children every material advantage. In reality, a strong undercurrent undermines parenthood. Social policies, media advertising, the Internet, social media, and societal norms make the already challenging job of being a competent parent more difficult. This reflects a deeply ingrained prejudice against individual children and childhood: juvenile ageism. This hidden prejudice, which is even more virulent than racism and sexism, makes it possible to ignore the well-being of our children and families.

If we really care about our children, asks David Lawrence, retired publisher of the Miami Herald, how is it that so many are treated so badly? (Miami Herald Staff 2012) Do we just not care? Are we not making the case coherently? Do we think we do not have the power to make people listen? Is it a lack of leadership? Lawrence points to all of these reasons, but if forced to select one, it would be the lack of leadership.

The intent of this book is to inspire leadership to ensure that all newborn babies in America have their most basic and essential requirement for an opportunity to succeed in life: parents who are able to raise them to become productive citizens. We can do this by applying the public health practices of primary, secondary, and tertiary prevention to child abuse and neglect. Primary prevention can be accomplished through life skills education in schools and by the small, but powerful, step of setting a simple, easily implemented standard for assuming the lifelong career of parenthood: a person under the custody of another person cannot assume the custody of another person—a newborn baby. Secondary prevention can be provided through home visitation programs for vulnerable families. Tertiary prevention can be implemented by extending the application of Child in Need of Protective Services to the prenatal stage.

References

Children's Defense Fund. (2007). America's cradle to prison pipeline. http://www.childrensdefense.org/library/data/cradle-prison-pipeline-report-2007-full-lowres.pdf. Accessed 7 July 2018.

Friedman, H. S. (2012). *The measure of a nation: How to regain America's competitive edge and boost our global standing*. New York: Prometheus Books.

Kennedy, R. F. (1968). Remarks at the University of Kansas, March 18, 1968. https://www.jfklibrary.org/Research/Research-Aids/Ready-Reference/RFK-Speeches/Remarks-of-Robert-F-Kennedy-at-the-University-of-Kansas-March-18-1968.aspx. Accessed 6 July 2018. Also found at https://images2.americanprogress.org/campus/email/RobertFKennedyUniversityofKansas.pdf. Accessed 6 July 2018.

Miami Herald Staff. (2012, July 9). David Lawrence Jr., early childhood education advocate, joining the University of Miami school of education. *Miami Herald*. http://www.miamiherald.com/news/local/education/article1941107.html. Accessed 7 July 2018.

Chapter 2
How Are Children in the United States Doing?

Never before have we subjected our children to the tyranny of drugs and guns and things or taught them to look for meaning outside rather than inside themselves, teaching them in Dr. King's words "to judge success by the value of our salaries or the size of our automobiles, rather than by the quality of our service and relationship to humanity."

Marian Wright Edelman, 1995, Children's Defense Fund
(Edelman 1995)

Most of our children and adolescents are doing well, but at least one in three is not as predicted by Marian Wright Edelman over 20 years ago. We should not be misled by rhetoric. We should not take comfort in downward trends in social problems, such as adolescent pregnancies or drug usage. We should not be misled by the image of parents who center their lives around their offspring. Those parents provide unprecedented levels of lessons, sports, tutoring, and camps, while over 15 million children and adolescents live in poverty (National Center for Children in Poverty). At least one in four children has experienced neglect and/or abuse at some point in their lives (CDC 2018a).

The growing gap in family wealth has created two sets of young people in the United States...those with educated, prosperous parents and those with less-educated, poor parents. As a result, most middle- and upper-class children and adolescents are thriving, while most lower-class children and adolescents are not. The backlash is evident in our unacceptable rates of child neglect and abuse, incarceration, homelessness, and welfare dependency.

If you are one of the American adults who live in a home without children—a majority these days—you need to know that the well-being of our nation's children affects you. Dire consequences arise when those of us without children miss the connection between the well-being of our young citizens and the wide-ranging social problems that affect all of us. We all must see the big picture...parents matter.

© Springer Nature Switzerland AG 2019
J. C. Westman, *Dealing with Child Abuse and Neglect as Public Health Problems*, https://doi.org/10.1007/978-3-030-05897-5_2

2.1   Hidden in Plain Sight

The daily news reports the myriad of ways in which many of our young are failing to the detriment of our society and our economy. Why does not this attract more public attention? Why do we not we make the connection between failing parents, failing children, and a failing society?

American politician, sociologist, and diplomat Daniel Patrick Moynihan gave an answer. He pointed out that societies, like individuals, cover up troublesome social problems with "painkillers" (Moynihan 1993–1994). He noted that the tolerance for deviant behavior increases over time. Deviancy is redefined in a way that excludes conduct we previously deplored. A prime example is homelessness. Intolerable in the United States 30 years ago, homelessness—even of families with children—is commonplace and accepted today.

Becoming numb to our social problems reflects our ability to adapt to stressful circumstances over which we believe we have no control. We become like the frog that fails to jump out of water heated so gradually that it allows itself to be cooked to death. We are being cooked by the plight of our young citizens and its impact on our society.

Measuring the well-being of our nation in economic terms like the gross domestic product (GDP)—the total value of goods and services produced—also allows us to avoid facing our social problems. In fact, costs associated with crime, disasters, and illness actually increase the GDP. Prisons enrich communities. Focusing only on the GDP blinds us to the health of our society and to the plight of our young people. We need better ways to accurately measure the well-being of our people (Fig. 2.1).

The Index of Social Health compiled by the Institute for Innovation in Social Policy at Vassar College measures the well-being of people. Sixteen social indicators are measured across all age groups. This index can be used to stimulate preventing rather than servicing our social and health problems.

Intriguingly, as our GDP has risen, the Index of Social Health has declined.

According to the latest data available from 1970 to 2011, 11 indicators have become worse:

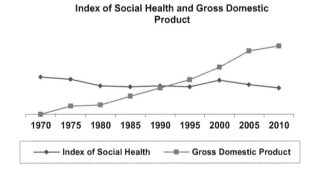

Fig. 2.1 Social health index and gross domestic product. (Source: Miringoff and Miringoff (1999). By permission of Oxford University Press, USA)

- Child poverty
- Income inequality
- Child abuse
- Teenage suicide
- Unemployment
- Average wages
- Health insurance coverage
- Out-of-pocket health-care costs for those 65 and older
- Food insecurity
- Access to affordable housing
- Homelessness

Seven indicators have improved, but this should not deter us from further improving them:

- Poverty among those 65 and older
- Infant mortality
- High school dropouts
- Teenage drug abuse
- Teenage pregnancies
- Homicides
- Alcohol-related traffic deaths

According to the Columbia University National Center for Children in Poverty, about 15 million children in the United States—21% of all children—lived in families with incomes below the federal poverty threshold in 2015. The Annie E. Casey Foundation's KIDS COUNT Data Book 2018 reported that 19% of children still were growing up in poverty. Research shows that, on average, families need an income of about twice that level to cover basic expenses. Using this standard, 43% of children live in low-income families (AEC 2018). The gulf continues to widen between children growing up in strong, economically secure families that are embedded in thriving communities and children who are not. While Black and Latino children continue to fall disproportionately into the latter group, large numbers of children of all racial and ethnic groups are facing economic conditions that can impede their long-term success.

Still, the latest data show continued incremental improvement in educational achievement and child health and safety, as well as a record low level of teen births, which has dropped 67% from 1991 to 2016, according to the National Center for Health Statistics (Hamilton et al. 2016). In 2016, the total number of US births was 3,941,109, a decline of 1% compared to 2015, a record low for the nation.

In spite of these improvements, the United States ranks 18th out of 21 Western countries in overall child well-being. Our children are clearly falling short intellectually. They rank 23rd in science, 17th in reading, and 31st in math achievement out of 32 Organization of Economic Cooperation and Development countries (National Center for Child Poverty). These include Shanghai, China (1st in all), Finland (1st, 2nd, and 6th), South Korea (6th, 2nd, and 4th), Canada (8th, 6th, and 10th), Germany

(13th, 20th, and 16th), and Poland (19th, 15th, and 25th). Martin Carnoy, professor of education at Stanford University, found that, when students with low socioeconomic status are removed, US students fare much better than international test comparisons suggest. This underscores the socioeconomic inequality between students in the United States.

Taken together along with unprecedented levels of school shootings, these conditions make the United States a leader among developed nations in signs of social distress. In his 1830s classic book *Democracy in America*, Alexis de Tocqueville observed that individualism had its roots in England (Lang 2005). From this comes his prediction for our time: economically developed English-speaking countries will have the highest levels of social and developmental disarray.

2.2   Growing Chaos for Our Youth

These statistics should not be surprising. Cornell University professor of human development Urie Bronfenbrenner, founder of the field of human ecology, called attention to the growing chaos in the lives of our children and adolescents 20 years ago, as did Marian Wright Edelman (SLJ 2011).

Since then we have seen:

- More children growing up in disadvantaged one-parent homes
- Increasing conflict between the demands of employment and family life
- Lack of positive adult role models
- Erosion of neighborhood ties between families
- Increasing divorced, step- and one-parent families
- A widening gap between the rich and the poor
- An increasing number of antisocial gangs
- Increasing numbers of school shootings

Another way to evaluate our society is by identifying and measuring the assets our young people need to develop and reach their full potential. The Search Institute's Developmental Assets framework has 2 groups of 20 assets: external and internal (Search Institute 1997).

The external assets are the positive experiences (social capital) young people receive in their lives. These assets identify the roles played by families, schools, congregations, neighborhoods, and youth organizations. The internal assets identify characteristics and behaviors (human capital) that reflect values, identities, and social competencies that promote a commitment to learning. Having 31 of all of the 40 external and internal assets is the desirable level. In 2010, only 6% of our adolescents had achieved that level. The average young person has only 20 assets, and boys have fewer than girls. Moreover, 37% of the young people surveyed reported being involved in two or more of the ten dangerous patterns of high-risk behavior studied.

In 2006, prior to the 2008 recession, a Gallup survey developed by Child Trends and the Search Institute reported that only 31% of America's children had all or most of the basic supports needed for healthy development: (1) caring adults, (2) safe places and constructive use of time, (3) healthy start in life and healthy development, (4) effective education for marketable skills and lifelong learning, and (5) opportunities to learn how to help others.

Both affluent and disadvantaged young people show evidence of the "syndrome of alienation" described by Bronfenbrenner: (1) inattentiveness and misbehavior in school; (2) academic underachievement; (3) smoking and drinking; (4) sexual activity; (5) alcohol and substance abuse; (6) dropping out of school; and ultimately (7) violence, crime, homicide, suicide, and welfare dependency.

Although genetic predisposition, pregnancy and birth complications, malnutrition, disabilities, poverty, and racism contribute to children's vulnerability, whether or not they show the "syndrome of alienation" largely depends on how they were parented. When parents are consumed by alcoholism, drug addiction, or mental disorders or when parents are preoccupied with personal interests or vocations and neglect and/or abuse their children, boys are prone to become criminals, while girls are prone to become welfare dependent through the Cradle to Prison/Welfare Dependency Pipeline.

Physically or emotionally absent parents are the common denominator in the record numbers of young people with psychiatric disorders, obesity, and sexually transmitted diseases. These problems cross class boundaries. In his book *The Vulnerable Child*, Richard Weissbourd concluded that the most serious threats to children—parental depression, a lack of meaningful opportunities, and social isolation—cut across class and race lines (Weissbourd 1997). Significantly, an increasing number of affluent parents place their offspring in therapeutic schools and programs like the 110 represented by the National Association of Therapeutic Schools and Programs.

2.3   Poverty

In 2015, 21% of all people under the age of 18—about 15 million—lived in poverty, four times the rate in Scandinavia. Blacks were at 38%, American Indians 35%, Latinos 32%, Asians 14%, and Whites 13%. The statistics for children living in families where no parent has full-time employment were Black 50%, American Indian 51%, Latino 39%, Asian 32%, and White 27%. Harry J. Holzer, professor of public policy at Georgetown University, estimated that the economic costs associated with childhood poverty total $500 billion a year (Power to Decide 2016).

2.3.1 Teen Pregnancy and Poverty

Poverty is both a cause and a consequence of teen pregnancy. One in four teen mothers will go on a welfare benefit program within 3 years of their child being born. Being a teen mother also means having less access to educational programs, which ultimately affects her ability to provide for the needs of her family later on in life.

Teen mothers are less likely to complete high school. They are much less likely to complete college. This puts them at a disadvantage when it comes time to find a good paying job. The evidence is clear. In the past two decades, the median income for college graduates has risen by 19%, while the median income for those who dropped out of high school has decreased by 28% (Vitanna Organization n.d.).

Yet, not all of the responsibility belongs to the mothers when it comes to teen pregnancy. Only one in five of the teen fathers of these children will go on to marry the mothers. This makes it essential for child support to be provided to maintain the stability of the household. Many teen fathers, however, pay less than $800 per year in child support because they do not have a good paying job.

Not only are teen fathers generally less educated themselves, but they experience earning losses that may exceed 15% each year. This creates a cycle of poverty which, if left unchecked, creates the likelihood for the next generation of children to deal with an unplanned pregnancy and to become teen parents.

2.3.2 Why Poverty Is a Factor in Teen Pregnancy

Education clearly is the one thing that can break the cycle of teen pregnancy. Yet, according to information from The National Campaign to Prevent Teen and Unplanned Pregnancy, this is exactly what teen mothers do not receive (Vitanna Organization n.d.).

- Eighty-nine percent of women who do not have a child as a teen will graduate from high school. Just 38% of teenage girls who have a child before the age of 18 will get a high school diploma by the age of 22.
- Thirty percent of teenage girls who decide to drop out of high school do so because of a pregnancy or giving birth.
- Two out of every three teen mothers who move out of their parents' home live below the poverty level.
- Less than 25% of teen mothers receive any child support payments from the fathers, which is why more than 60% receive some sort of public benefit before their children's first birthdays.

Poverty has a negative effect on the children born into these situations as well. When a child is born to a mother who is younger than 18, that child has a higher risk of scoring "significantly worse" on school readiness exams that include math and reading. This struggle creates an intergenerational complication which encourages poverty because there is an overall lack of resources available in teen households.

Poverty matters because it can be the cause of teen pregnancy, while teen pregnancy also can be the cause of poverty. This means we need to intervene when a pregnancy happens so that the teens involved can get back on their feet from an educational standpoint. As Martha Kempner writes for Rewire: "Let's face it: if you graduate from high school and get a job, you are two steps ahead when it comes to not living in poverty, whether or not you get married and have kids" (OJJDP 2017).

2.3.3   Why Does Poverty Actually Cause Teen Pregnancies?

Interestingly enough, the cause of many teen pregnancies is that young women are choosing to become mothers at an early age. It is more than just teens being trapped in a cycle of poverty or having some households treating a teen pregnancy as a cultural norm. It is because there is a conscious, logical assessment of the teen's future potential in society and that evaluation leads girls in particular to decide to become parents. If teen girls feel like their chances of being economically successful are low, even if they do their best to do everything in the "right way," then their choice, more often than not, is to embrace the idea of becoming a teen parent and having a baby to love them. The reason for this is basic satisfaction. The feeling of being a parent, especially at first, can be incredibly gratifying. Teens choose this gratification despite the fact that financial, educational, and employment opportunities are few and far between for them.

2.4   Crime

According to the Office of Juvenile Justice and Delinquency Prevention, the juvenile arrest rate for all offenses reached its highest level in the last three decades in 1996 and then declined 70% by 2016. Still, adolescents and young adults are victims of violent crime at the highest rates (Hawkins 2012).

Homicide rates for US males ages 15 through 24 are more than four times those in other developed countries. Juvenile crime is rising in the form of violence by girls in gangs. A decade ago, the ratio in arrests for assaults between boys and girls was ten to one. Now the ratio is four to one.

While violent crime has reached historic lows in cities like New York, Miami, and Los Angeles, it is rising sharply in Milwaukee and other cities across the nation. Violent crime is expected to increase over the next decade as more violent felons are released from prisons without effective rehabilitation programs for them.

In the 1990s, homicides largely occurred in gang battles over drug turfs. Now they happen over petty disputes. In Milwaukee, a woman killed a friend during an argument over a silk dress. A man killed a neighbor whose 10-year-old son had mistakenly used his soap. Two men argued over a cell phone, pulled out their guns, and killed a 13-year-old girl in the crossfire. Milwaukee Police Chief Nannette Hegerty called it "the rage thing." We're seeing a very angry population, and they don't go to fists anymore; they go right to guns.

The typical characteristics of adolescent crimes are demonstrated in shocking yet not uncommon examples. Five bored teenagers used Molotov cocktails to set fire to 14 vehicles and 1 house. They took police on a tour of the arson spree and implicated themselves in three earlier house fires. Police said, "It was like show-and-tell."

Eighteen-year-old Sarah Rose Ludemann was stabbed to death by 19-year-old Rachel Marie Wade. According to a witness, Wade plunged a kitchen knife into Ludemann's heart. The two had been at odds over their on-again, off-again boyfriend, a 19-year-old who had fathered a child with a third woman.

In Hillsborough County, Florida, sheriff's deputies arrested a 15-year-old and three 14-year-olds who violated a 13-year-old with a broom handle and a hockey stick in a locker room at Walker Middle School.

A dispute between two boys at a high school in an affluent suburb of Miami left one dead from a knife wound. A 14-year-old boy stabbed his best friend to death at a South Florida middle school. A handful of shootings and stabbings have occurred at schools in that area, although no one was killed.

In Chicago, more than 440 school-age children were shot in 2012; 60 died (Hess 2006). "I think people in Chicago have almost gotten numb to the statistics," said Dexter Voisin, a researcher at the University of Chicago. "For every kid who is murdered, about 100 kids witness a murder or are victims of nonfatal injuries, robberies, muggings and gang-related incidents."

The ready availability of assault weapons has enabled angry young men to create havoc in schools.

2.5   Behavior Problems in Schools

In a 2006 AP-AOL Learning Services Poll, two-thirds of the teachers surveyed said student discipline and lack of interest are major problems. School bus drivers must deal with disrespectful and unruly riders. There is a national trend for young teachers to leave within 1–3 years. Increasingly, we are seeing reports such that from the Columbus Mississippi Municipal School District where 49% of employees who responded to an anonymous employee survey in 2016 reported they would not recommend the district as a place to work (Altman 2017).

Even in the late 1990s, 47% of 3500 kindergarten teachers surveyed said that at least half their students had problems following directions. Some of the issues were due to poor academic skills, while others came from difficulties working in a group. When presented with the statement that an atmosphere of respect, trust, and pride toward adults existed in their schools in a 2008 Pinellas County, Florida, survey, 37% of teachers disagreed. In Milwaukee public schools, the number was 25%. Among students, it was 49%.

In 2015 in the relatively prosperous Madison Metropolitan School District (n.d.), 13% of the students and 42% of the teachers felt that parents were not helping them succeed. Among students, 22% felt they would not get into trouble at home if they breeched school rules; 25% felt unsafe at school; 60% felt that their personal possessions were unsafe at school; 61% felt vulnerable to bullying; 54% felt vulnerable to sexual harassment; and 45% felt they could not talk with an adult at school about drugs, sex, or suicidal comments made by other students.

Thirty years ago, the disciplinary problems found in schools involved chewing gum, stepping out of line, tardiness, and occasional fist fights. Today they include attacks on teachers, rape in the hallways, murder, and suicide. From 1992 to 2006, over 400 murders occurred at lower-class urban schools, and 33 shootings took place in middle-class schools. Many more deaths have been averted since then by early responses to warning signals. Children continue to shoot children but shootings no longer merit significant media attention. Since the Columbine shooting in 1999, there have been 19 school shootings. The following are examples:

- A 7-year-old boy shot a 5-year-old three times. It was reported in the second section of the St. Petersburg Times.
- Seventeen-, 16-, and 13-year-olds talked about how a fight would be fun and then stabbed a 34-year-old man to death.
- An 18-year-old Cape Cod Regional Technical High School student threatened to blow up the school with a pipe bomb he had made.
- A 15-year-old boy in Clearwater, Florida, said he wanted to do something like the Columbine school shootings. In his room was a small arsenal together with videos of the shootings, executions, and images of the president and vice president as targets.
- Two 17-year-old boys in Green Bay, Wisconsin, had weapons and bombs. They intended to repeat the Columbine shootings.
- In February 2012, a school shooting in Chardon, Ohio, did receive national attention as did the December 2012 shooting in Newton, Connecticut.
- In February 2018, a teen gunman opened fire with a semiautomatic rifle at his former high school in Parkland, Florida, killing 17 people.

Although there is no typical mental illness profile of school shooters, they consistently report that they had no adults with whom they could talk, including their own parents. A growing number of teenagers are uncontrollable and unreachable because they did not form stable attachment bonds with their parents. Since they do not have effective consciences, they become drug addicts, thieves, rapists, and murderers. Many were disadvantaged at birth by cocaine withdrawal or premature births and experienced frightening, insecure infancies. Their neglectful, often drug-using parents were unable to provide for their needs.

Bullying has reached unprecedented levels in our schools with suicide as a possible consequence. According to the *Family and Work Institute*, cited by the National Crime Prevention Council (n.d.), one-third of youth are bullied at least once a month, while others say six out of ten American teens witness bullying at least once a day. Witnessing bullying can be harmful as it makes witnesses feel helpless or that they may be the next target. In a study by *Fight Crime: Invest in Kids*, nearly 60%

of boys classified as bullies in grades 6–9 were convicted of at least one crime by the age of 24, while 40% had three or more convictions.

2.6   The Achievement Gap

According to the National Center for Education Statistics, in school year 2014–2015, the adjusted cohort graduation rate (ACGR) for public high school students rose to 83% in the United States, the highest rate since the measure was first reported in 2010–2011. Asian/Pacific Islander students had the highest ACGR (90%), followed by White (88%), Hispanic (78%), Black (75%), and American Indian/Alaska Native (72%) students (NCES 2018).

Still, we must find a solution for what Professor Robert Balfanz of Johns Hopkins University calls our "dropout factories" (Watts 2011). At 12% of high schools (about 2000), graduation is at best a 50/50 proposition. About 23% of young Black male dropouts are incarcerated compared to a rate of 6–7% for Asians, Hispanics, and Whites. Female school dropouts are more than six times as likely to give birth and nearly nine times as likely to become single mothers when compared to peers who attended college.

The Program for International Student Assessment reported that in 2015 average scores of 15-year-olds in science literacy ranged from 556 in Singapore to 332 in the Dominican Republic (OECD 2018). The US average score was 496 similar to the overall average of 493. The US average was lower than 18 education systems, higher than 39, and not measurably different than 12.

According to the 2018 Kids Count Report (Annie E. Casey Foundation 2018), an alarming 65% of fourth graders in public school were reading below the proficient level in 2017, a slight improvement from 2007, when the figure was 68%. State differences in fourth-grade reading levels among public school students were wide. In 2015, Massachusetts had the lowest percentage of public school fourth graders not proficient in reading, 50%, compared with a high of 77% in New Mexico. The percentage of high school graduates who entered college were 66% for Asians, 47% for Whites, 40% for Blacks, and 32% for Latinos.

Since 2010, the GradNation campaign has focused the nation's attention and the work of America's Promise Alliance on raising national graduation rates to 90% by 2020 while dramatically increasing postsecondary career training or college enrollment and completion.

The percentage of students who graduate from community public college campuses within 6 years generally ranges from 17% to 58% (Ross et al. 2012). Twenty percent of college students completing 4-year degrees and 30% of students earning 2-year degrees have only basic literacy and math skills. In an American Institute for Research study, they were unable to estimate whether their car had enough gasoline to reach the next station or calculate the total cost for a variety of office supplies.

2.7 Mental Health

In 2001, Surgeon General David Satcher released the National Action Agenda for Children's Mental Health in response to the crisis in mental health care for children and adolescents (Suttenfield 2001). At that time, 10% suffered from severe mental illnesses, yet only one in five received mental health services. Satcher's declared crisis has worsened. According to the National Alliance on Mental Health, in 2016, 20% of young people had been diagnosed with a psychiatric disorder by the age of 18.

The Centers for Disease Control's 2016 Youth Risk Behavior Survey (YRBS) revealed that significant progress has been made in reducing physical fighting among adolescents (CDC 2018b). Since 1991, the percentage of high school students who had been in a physical fight at least once during the past 12 months decreased from 42% to 23%. However, in 2016, nationwide the percentage of students who had not gone to school because of safety concerns was still too high, with 6% of students missing at least 1 day of school during the past month because they felt they would be unsafe. The YRBS noted that two-thirds of adolescents receive too little sleep, a condition that increases behaviors that are harmful to a person's well-being.

The World Health Organization indicates that by the year 2020, childhood psychiatric disorders will rise by over 50% (WHO 2001). They will become one of the five most common causes of morbidity, mortality, and disability among children. The lack of a unified mental health infrastructure in the United States allows many of these children to fall through the cracks. Too often, children whose mental health problems go unnoticed as well as those with recognized but untreated ailments end up in prison.

Our educational and health-care systems do not sufficiently help adolescents develop healthy routines, behaviors, and relationships they can carry into their adult lives. While most are doing reasonably well, most adolescents who need them do not have access to mental health and substance abuse services. Others engage in risky behaviors that jeopardize their current health and contribute to poor health in adulthood. Children and families suffer because of missed opportunities for the prevention and early identification of problems and because of fragmented services.

2.8 Alcohol Abuse, Drug Abuse, and Smoking

The National Longitudinal Study of Adolescent to Adult Health found in 2008 that suburban high school students drink, smoke, use illegal drugs, and are engaged in delinquent behavior as often or more than urban high school students (Cheng et al. 2015).

- Sixty-three percent of suburban and 57% of urban 12th graders drank when away from family members.

- Forty percent of 12th graders in both urban and suburban schools had used illegal drugs.
- Thirty-seven percent of suburban 12th graders have smoked at least once a day compared to 30% of urban 12th graders.
- Urban and suburban students were equally likely to fight and steal.
- Half of all adolescents attended parties where drugs and alcohol were available. One-third attended a party where alcohol, marijuana, cocaine, ecstasy, or prescription drugs were available, while a parent was present.
- Underage drinking accounted for at least 16% of alcohol sales in 2001. Every year, some 5000 young people under the age of 21 die as a result of drinking. This number includes deaths from motor vehicle crashes, homicides, suicide, and other injuries such as falls, burns, and drowning.

According to the University of Michigan Monitoring the Future National Survey (MFNS) in 2017, alcohol remains the substance most widely used by today's teenagers (Johnson et al. 2017). Despite recent declines, two out of every three students have consumed alcohol more than just a few sips by the end of high school, and over a quarter have done so by the 8th grade. In fact, half of 12th graders and one in nine 8th graders reported having been drunk at least once in their life. The estimated abuse rates for illegal drugs other than marijuana were 3.4% in the 8th, 5.4% in the 10th, and 9% in the 12th grades.

About 90% of smokers begin before they turn 21. According to the MFNS, the prevalence of cigarette use continued its long-term decline in 2014 in all three grades: to 14% in the 8th grade, to 23% in the 10th grade, and to 34% in the 12th grade. The 2016 Youth Risk Behavior Survey found that 24% of high school students reported using e-cigarettes (Johnson et al. 2017). Most said they would like to quit but were unable to do so. Cigarette smoking during childhood and adolescence produces significant health problems including respiratory illnesses, diminished physical fitness, and retarded lung growth.

Adolescents use illicit drugs for recreation and prescription drugs for specific effects. Stimulants help them study, sedatives bring sleep, and tranquilizers relieve stress. The 2016 National Survey on Drug Use and Health (NSDUH) reported that the abuse of prescription drugs is highest among young adults ages 18–25, with 5.9% reporting nonmedical use in the past month (SAMSHA 2016). Among youth ages 12–17, 3% reported past-month nonmedical use of prescription medications. Nearly one-third believed there was nothing wrong with using prescription medicines once in a while; they also believed that prescription pain relievers were not addictive.

According to the NSDUH, 12.8% of adolescents ages 12–17 and 10.9% of young adults ages 18–25 had a major depressive episode (MDE) during the past year. The percentage of adolescents ages 12–17 who had a substance use disorder (SUD) in the past year was higher among those with a past-year MDE than it was among those without it (31.7% vs. 13.4%). An estimated 333,000 adolescents (1.4% of all adolescents) had both an SUD and an MDE in the past year. 71.9% of them received either substance use treatment at a specialty facility or mental health service in the past year.

2.9   Adolescent Sexually Transmitted Diseases

The 2016 Youth Risk Behavior Survey showed mixed results regarding youth sexual risk behaviors (CDC 2018c). While teens are having less sex, condom use among currently sexually active students and HIV testing among all students have declined. The percentage of high school students who had sexual intercourse during the past 3 months has decreased from 38% in 1991 to 30% in 2015. However, among high school students who are currently sexually active, condom use declined from 63% in 2003 to 57% in 2015.

According to the Centers for Disease Control and Prevention, about four million or one in four sexually active adolescent girls and boys (48% of Black youth and 20% of White youth) contracts a sexually transmitted disease (CDC 2018b). Of the some 900,000 adolescents who run away from home each year, over 6% test positive for the AIDS virus. Each year up to 64,000 adolescents spread AIDS.

Adolescent sexually transmitted disease rates are much higher in the United States than in most other developed countries. Rates are ten times higher for syphilis and gonorrhea and two to five times higher for chlamydia. Although the age of sexual debut varies little across countries, American adolescents are the most likely to have multiple partners. The younger the sexual debut, the more likely health hazards become.

2.10   Adolescent Childbirth

Adolescent childbirth is an international issue. Former President Bill Clinton wants to empower women to reduce birth rates because population growth is a major contributor to global warming. He calls for "slowing the population explosion in countries that can't take care of the people they have now."

Adolescent birth rates in the United States along with Bulgaria and Romania are the highest of developed nations. This is in part the result of the greater number of sexual partners among adolescents (Martin et al. 2017) (Fig. 2.2).

In 2015, the birth rate for girls ages 10–14 was 0.2/1000, meaning that of some 10 million girls, 2012 gave birth (Fig. 2.3).

There were 24.2 births for every 1000 adolescent females ages 15–19, or 249,078 babies born to females in this age group. Nearly 89% of these births occurred outside of marriage. Although Black and Hispanic girls are more than twice as likely as White girls to become pregnant at least once before the age of 20, the actual births to White girls far exceed those to them. Of the 251,090 births to 10- to 19-year-old girls, an estimated 238,903 were White; 41,142 were Latino; and 32,631 were Black.

From 1990 to 2002, the pregnancy rate for girls ages 15–19 dropped from 111 to 76/1000, a record low. This continuing trend indicates an increased motivation to avoid pregnancies possibly influenced by reduced incentives to give birth

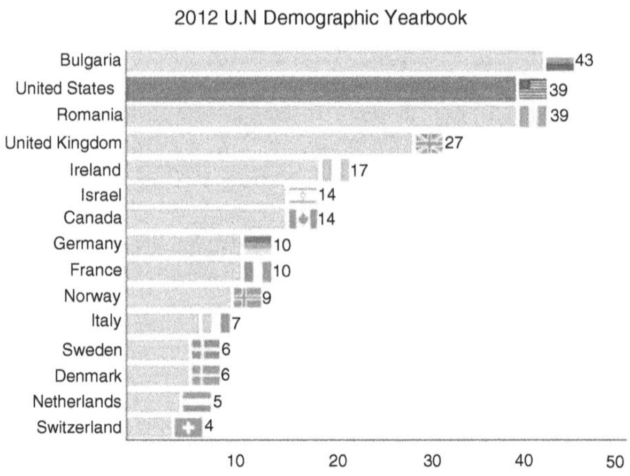

2012 U.N Demographic Yearbook

Fig. 2.2 Teen birth rates. (Source: Centers for Disease Control and Prevention (CDC), Division of Reproductive Health, National Center for Chronic Disease Prevention and Health Promotion. (2015). Birth rates (live births) per 1,000 females aged 15–19 years, by race and Hispanic ethnicity, select years. Centers for Disease Control and Prevention (CDC). https://www.cdc.gov/teenpregnancy/about/birth-rates-chart-2000-2011-text.htm. Accessed 2 August 2018)

through more restrictive access to welfare benefits in the Temporary Assistance for Needy Families program under the Personal Responsibility and Work Opportunity Act of 1996.

Over 2.5 million of our children and adolescents have been born to mothers under the age of 18. Almost a third of all sexually experienced adolescent girls have been pregnant. An estimated 22% of Black, 19% of Latino, and 10% of White teenage boys have impregnated a girl. These figures are low since males might not always be informed about partners' miscarriages or terminations.

Adolescents ages 15 through 19 account for one-third of all unwed mothers. As mentioned before, up to one-third of 15- to 19-year-olds' births result from desired pregnancies. Over one-third of these mothers become pregnant again within 18 months. Most fail to return to school and become dependent on welfare. Less than 2% of mothers who have a baby before the age of 18 finish college by age 30. A substitute teacher in a New York high school made the following observation:

> I hear talk about becoming pregnant on purpose. I watch the girls who are pregnant become the center of attention, watch them feel important. I watch boys brag about the babies they've fathered as proof of their masculinity and see girls emotionally attach to boys like to the father they never had.

In the 1960s, adolescent childbearing occurred mostly in marriage with an employed husband. Now it is with unwed adolescents with limited prospects of marriage and economic security.

A National Campaign to Prevent Teen and Unplanned Pregnancy survey found that a majority of adolescent parents came from households that were not in poverty and that were not headed by single parents (NCSL 2018). However, a dispro-

U.S. Birth Rates for Teens 15-19 Years by Race/Ethnicity, 1991 and 2009

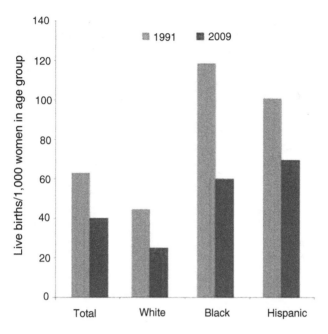

Fig. 2.3   Teen birth rates by race and ethnicity. (Source: Centers for Disease Control and Prevention (CDC), Division of Reproductive Health, National Center for Chronic Disease Prevention and Health Promotion, & National Center for Health Statistics, Division of Vital Statistics. (2011). Vital signs: teen pregnancy – United States, 1991 – 2009. *Morbidity and Mortality Weekly Report (MMWR)*. Centers for Disease Control and Prevention (CDC). https://www.cdc.gov/mmwr/preview/mmwrhtml/mm6013a5.htm. Accessed 2 August 2018)

portionate share comes from households with incomes either below or just above poverty levels as well as from households lacking one or both biological parents. The conception rate for boys is lower than the birth rate for girls because 39% of the fathers of children born to 15-year-olds and 47% of the fathers of children born to 16-year-olds are older than 20.

2.11   Other Risks

According to the Centers for Disease Control and Prevention, motor vehicle crashes are the leading cause of death among American teenagers (CDC 2017). They killed 2700 teenagers in 2010, a greater number than homicides and suicides. The accident rate among 16- to 19-year-olds is three times that of older drivers.

According to GASP, an educational campaign organized by parents of victims of the "choking game," 17-year-old Macklin Jensen died while participating in the game in which adolescents strangle themselves or have others push on their chests so they can feel lightheaded for a few seconds (Schultz 2009).

Each one of us carries at least 250 toxic chemicals in our bodies. The young are the most vulnerable to their damaging effects. *Pediatric Environmental Health* highlights lead, mercury, PCBs, and pesticide poisoning as known hazards to children's health (AAP 2012). **Numerous studies confirm that even slightly elevated lead levels in the blood can cause learning and behavioral disorders, decreased IQ, and hearing impairments. Many environmental chemicals mimic hormones that can disrupt developing immune, nervous,** and endocrine systems. The greatest vulnerability to toxic chemicals occurs during pregnancy.

All of these chemical hazards are at their highest levels in the environments of disadvantaged, pregnant adolescents. Efforts to make manufacturers demonstrate that chemicals released into the environment are not hazardous to the health of children largely have been unsuccessful. This is in part because the thresholds for deaths from lead, PCB, or mercury exposure are much higher than for altered cognitive and behavioral development. A disease-like cancer also is more readily perceived as "real" than failing school performance.

Overall child deaths in the United States greatly exceed those in comparable nations, largely because of the prevalence of gun shootings (Table 2.1).

Table 2.1 Child death rates, 2017

Child deaths, 2017	
Thousands of annual deaths per one million children, up through age 19	
United States	6.5
Canada	5.2
United Kingdom	4.6
Australia	4.3
Average	4.8
France	3.8
Germany	3.6
Italy	3.3
Spain	3.3
Sweden	2.7
Japan	2.5

Source: United Nations Inter-agency Group for Child Mortality Estimation (UN IGME). (2017). Levels & trends in child mortality: report 2017, estimates developed by the UN Inter-agency Group for Child Mortality Estimation. United Nations Inter-agency Group for Child Mortality Estimation (UN IGME). https://www.unicef.org/publications/files/Child_Mortality_Report_2017.pdf. Accessed 2 August 2018
Average covers 20 high-income nations that are members of the OECD. See: Thakrar et al. (2018)

2.12 Steeped in Social Toxins

In 1979, I estimated that 16% of our children had significant physical, developmental, mental, educational, and social problems. Even more strikingly, 37% of our children were thought to be at risk for maladjustment. The intervening years have borne out that forecast. Combining the following demographics indicates that at least one-third of our young people under the age of 19 (some 24 million) have educational, health, mental health, behavioral, or economic problems that impair the quality of their lives.

James Garbarino, professor of psychology at Loyola University-Chicago, stands with developmental psychologist Urie Bronfenbrenner who described our "socially toxic environment" that has created a larger number of children with serious problems today than was seen in the 1950s and 1960s. "Social contaminants" include exposure to violence, economic pressure, disrupted family relationships, and behaviors stemming from depression, paranoia, bullying, and alienation.

These social contaminants demoralize families and communities. The American Academy of Pediatrics confirmed this conclusion in its 2012 Policy Statement Early Childhood Adversity, Toxic Stress, and the Role of the Pediatrician: Translating Developmental Science into Lifelong Health (APA 2012). The Academy develops innovative strategies to reduce the effects of toxic stress in young children as well as negative effects on development and health across the entire life span (Table 2.2).

William Julius Wilson, professor of sociology at Harvard University, points out that both societal and cultural impediments keep poor Blacks from escaping poverty (Schorow 2008). Three generations of Black ghetto dwellers have relied on sporadic work and welfare. Isolated in their urban neighborhoods, they have almost no contact with mainstream American society or the typical job market. As a result, they have distinctive and often dysfunctional social norms. A work ethic, investment in the future, and deferred gratification make no sense when legitimate employment at a living wage does not exist and when crime is both an everyday hazard and temptation. Men unable to support their families abandon them; women resign themselves to single motherhood and the status and benefits it accords; and children suffer from broken homes and antisocial examples set by peers and adults. This dysfunctional behavior reinforces negative racial stereotypes, making it all the more difficult for poor Blacks to find decent jobs.

We cannot expect our children to prosper when our society does not value and even undermines character development. The good life is portrayed as having power, pleasure, and possessions…gained by any means as described by Benjamin Barber in his book *Consumed*. Little emphasis is placed on the strength of character needed to control one's impulses, to tolerate frustration, and to postpone gratification—all essential for life in a civilized society. Children are not born with these qualities. They learn them from adults. They learn them most indelibly from competent parents in a social environment that supports parenthood.

The child psychiatrist Harold Kopelwicz described "affluenza" as an illness contracted when people measure their worth with material goods. Children with this

Table 2.2 Indicators of children and youth well-being

Indicators of children and youth well-being	
Categories of persons under 19	Percentage
Living in poverty	22%
Did not graduate from high school on time	22%
Have a diagnosed mental disorder (Keyes 2006)	20%
Substantiated victims of child maltreatment (ACF 2009)	15%
In child welfare, juvenile justice, or homeless/runaway systems (ages 12–19) (Perper and Manlove 2009)	23%
Fourth graders not proficient in reading	68%
Eighth-graders not proficient in math	66%
Twelfth-graders who smoke once a day (Child Trends (2012)	10%
Binge drink (Eaton et al. 2012)	22%
Use illegal drugs (SAMHSA 2012)	10%
Abuse medications (ages 15–19) (OAS 2008)	20%
Sexually transmitted diseases (ages 15–19) (Weinstock et al. 2004)	13%
Rated as not flourishing in mental health (ages 15–19) (Keyes 2006)	60%
No parent has full-time employment (2010)	33%
Children who are or have lived in one-parent homes (Gottlieb 2005)	50%
Personal assets: (Benson et al. 2011)	
Positive self-esteem	52%
Integrity	71%
Achievement motivation	71%
Delay gratification	50%
Positive peer influence	68%

illness lack resilience (Koplewicz et al. 2009). They have little patience or problem-solving abilities; they do not understand cause and effect; and they lack independence in following through on tasks.

2.13 The Way It Is

The growing discrepancy in family wealth has created two sets of young people: those with educated, thriving parents and those with less-educated, poor parents. Only 31% of our children have all of the five basic supports thought to be needed for optimal healthy development. One-third have significant educational, health, mental health, or behavioral problems. Disruptive behavior in many schools necessitates the presence of police.

An increasing cohort of children is growing up uncontrollable and unreachable because they did not form secure attachment bonds during early life. They do not have functioning consciences. As our physical and social environments become more toxic, our young show the effects first as well as the most.

Our society appears to need delinquents and criminals to act out the hidden impulses we gratify through violent, sexually stimulating media. We then subject offenders to indignant censure. In this sense, the "badness" of delinquents and criminals gratifies our own impulses. By punishing others, we can avoid facing our own "badness."

We need to strengthen struggling families in order to prevent antisocial behavior. Instead, we expect schools and governmental agencies to correct our social problems, as if parents have nothing to do with the outcomes of their children's lives.

We can and must remove the barriers to developing a responsible, productive citizenry by helping the families of over 15 million young people find pathways out of poverty. We also must address the needs of over 11 million children and youth who have been damaged by neglect or abuse. When we elevate the bar of tolerable deviant behavior, we clearly denigrate our youngest citizens and their parents.

References

AAP [American Academy of Pediatrics Council on Environmental Health]. (2012). In R.A. Etzel, & S.J. Balk (Eds.), *Pediatric environmental health*, 3rd ed. Elk Grove Village, IL: American Academy of Pediatrics.

ACF [Administration on Children, Youth, and Families]. (2009). *Child maltreatment 2009*. Washington, DC: Government Printing Office. https://www.acf.hhs.gov/archive/cb/resource/child-maltreatment-2009. Accessed 6 July 2018.

Altman, I. (2017, October 11). Student discipline cited as reason teachers are leaving CMSD. *The Dispatch* [Columbus and Starkville, Mississippi]. http://www.cdispatch.com/news/article.asp?aid=61268. Accessed 6 July 2018.

Annie E. Casey Foundation. (2018). KIDS COUNT data book, state trends in child well-being. https://www.aecf.org/resources/2018-kids-count-data-book/. Accessed 21 Sept 2018.

APA [American Pediatric Association]. (2012). Early childhood adversity, toxic stress, and the role of the pediatrician: Translating developmental science into lifelong health. *Pediatrics, 129*(1), e224–e231. https://doi.org/10.1542/peds.2011-2662. http://pediatrics.aappublications.org/content/129/1/e224. Accessed 6 July 2018.

Benson, P. L., Scales, P. C., Roehlkepartain, E. C., & Leffert, N. (2011). *A fragile foundation: The state of developmental assets among American youth*. Minneapolis: Search Institute.

CDC [Centers for Disease Control and Prevention]. (2017). *Teen drivers: Get the facts*. Centers for Disease Control and Prevention. https://www.cdc.gov/motorvehiclesafety/teen_drivers/teendrivers_factsheet.html. Accessed 6 July 2018.

CDC [Centers for Disease Control and Prevention]. (2018a). Child abuse and neglect: Consequences. https://www.cdc.gov/violenceprevention/childabuseandneglect/consequences.html. Accessed 6 July 2018.

CDC [Centers for Disease Control and Prevention]. (2018b). CDC releases youth risk behaviors survey results. https://www.cdc.gov/features/yrbs/index.html. Accessed 6 July 2018.

CDC [Centers for Disease Control and Prevention]. (2018c). *Sexual risk behaviors: HIV, STD, & teen pregnancy prevention*. CDC. https://www.cdc.gov/healthyyouth/sexualbehaviors/. Accessed 6 July 2018.

Cheng, W., et al. (2015). Alcohol use among adolescent youth: The role of friendship networks and family factors in multiple school studies. *PLoS One, 10*(3), e0119965. https://www.ncbi.nlm.nih.gov/pmc/articles/PMC4355410/. Accessed 6 July 2018.

Child Trends. (2012). Child trends data bank. https://www.childtrends.org/. Accessed 6 July 2018.

Eaton, D. K., Kann, L., Kinchen, S. A., et al. (2012). Youth risk behavior surveillance—United States, 2011. *CDC Morbidity Mortality Surveillance Summary, 61*(SS-04), 1–162.

Gottlieb, L. (2005). The XY files. *The Atlantic, 296*(2), 141–150. https://www.theatlantic.com/magazine/archive/2005/09/the-xy-files/304172/. Accessed 6 July 2018.

Hamilton, B. E., Rossen, L. M., & Branum, A. M. (2016). *Teen birth rates for urban and rural areas in the United States, 2007–2015* (NCHS data brief, no 264). Hyattsville: National Center for Health Statistics. https://www.cdc.gov/nchs/products/databriefs/db264.htm. Accessed 6 July 2018.

Hawkins, A. (2012). 440+ school age children shot in gun-controlled Chicago. http://www.breitbart.com/big-government/2012/12/24/chicago-is-gun-control-capital-of-u-s-yet-over-440-school-age-children-shot-there-in-2012/. Accessed 6 July 2018.

Hess, F. (2006, May). What to think, not how to think. *Education Matters*. https://www.aaeteachers.org/newsletters/maynews06.pdf. Accessed 6 July 2018.

Johnston, L. D., O'Malley, P. M., Miech, R. A., Bachman, J. G., & Schulenberg, J. E. (2017). *Monitoring the future national survey results on drug use, 1975–2016: Overview, key findings on adolescent drug use*. Ann Arbor: Institute for Social Research, The University of Michigan. http://www.monitoringthefuture.org/pubs/monographs/mtf-overview2016.pdf. Accessed 6 July 2018.

Keyes, C. L. M. (2006). Mental health in adolescence. *American Journal of Orthopsychiatry, 76*(3), 395–402.

Kopelwicz, H. S., Gurian, A., & Williams, K. (2009). The era of affluence and its discontents. *Journal of the Academy of Child and Adolescent Psychiatry, 48*(11), 1053–1055.

Lang, S. (2005, September 26). Urie Bronfenbrenner, father of Head Start program and pre-eminent 'human ecologist,' dies at age 88. *Cornell Chronicle*. http://news.cornell.edu/stories/2005/09/head-start-founder-urie-bronfenbrenner-dies-88. Accessed 6 July 2018.

Madison Metropolitan School District. (n.d.). https://www.madison.k12.wi.us/majorgrowth. Accessed 6 July 2018.

Martin, J. A., Hamilton, B., et al. (2017). Births: Final data for 2015. *National Vital Statistics Reports, 66*(1). https://www.cdc.gov/nchs/data/nvsr/nvsr66/nvsr66_01.pdf. Accessed 6 July 2018.

Miringoff, M., & Miringoff, M. L. (1999). *The social health of the nation: How America is really doing*. Oxford: Oxford University Press.

Moynihan, D. P. (1993–1994). Defining deviancy down: How we've become accustomed to alarming levels of crime and destructive behavior. *American Educator*. https://timemilitary.files.wordpress.com/2012/03/defining-deviancy-down-amereducator.pdf. Accessed 6 July 2018.

National Crime Prevention Council. (n.d.). Bullying. http://archive.ncpc.org/topics/bullying.html. Accessed 6 July 2018.

NCES [National Center for Education Statistics]. (2018). Public high school graduation rates. (Last Updated: May 2018). https://nces.ed.gov/programs/coe/indicator_coi.asp. Accessed 6 July 2018.

NCSL [National Conference of State Legislatures]. (2018). Teen pregnancy intervention. http://www.ncsl.org/research/health/teen-pregnancy-prevention.aspx. Accessed 6 July 2018.

OAS [Office of Applied Studies]. (2008). *The NSDUH report: Misuse of over-the-counter cough and cold medications among persons aged 12–25*. Rockville: SAMHS. http://homelesshub.ca/resource/misuse-over-counter-cough-and-cold-medications-among-persons-aged-12-25. Accessed 6 July 2018.

OECD [Organisation for Economic Co-operation and Development]. (2018). PISA 2015 results in focus. https://www.oecd.org/pisa/pisa-2015-results-in-focus.pdf. Accessed 6 July 2018.

OJJDP [Office of Juvenile Justice and Delinquency Prevention]. (2017). Department of Justice statistical briefing book, Juvenile Arrest Rate Trends. https://www.ojjdp.gov/ojstatbb/crime/JAR_Display.asp. Accessed 6 July 2018.

Perper, K., & Manlove, J. (2009). *Vulnerable youth: A closer look at reproductive outcomes. Putting what works to work September*. Washington, DC: Child Trends.

Power to Decide. (2016). Teen pregnancy national data. https://powertodecide.org/what-we-do/information/national-state-data/national. Accessed 6 July 2018.

Ross, T., Kena, G., Rathbun, A., Kewal Ramani, A., Zhang, J., Kristapovich, P., & Manning, E. (2012). *Higher education: Gaps in access and persistence study (NCES 2012-046). U.S. Department of Education, National Center for Education Statistics.* Washington, DC: Government Printing Office. https://nces.ed.gov/pubs2012/2012046.pdf. Accessed 6 July 2018.

SAMHSA [Substance Abuse and Mental Health Services Administration]. (2012). Results from the 2011 National survey on drug use and health: Summary of national findings. NSDUH Series H-44, HHS Publication No. (SMA) 12-4713. https://www.samhsa.gov/data/sites/default/files/NSDUHresults2012/NSDUHresults2012.pdf. Accessed 6 July 2018.

SAMHSA [Substance Abuse and Mental Health Services Administration]. (2016). Reports and detailed tables from the 2016 National Survey on Drug Use and Health (NSDUH). https://www.samhsa.gov/samhsa-data-outcomes-quality/major-data-collections/reports-detailed-tables-2016-NSDUH. Accessed 6 July 2018.

Schorow, S. (2008). Wilson perceives social structure and culture as key causes of poverty. *The Harvard Gazette*, October 9. https://news.harvard.edu/gazette/story/2008/10/wilson-perceives-social-structure-and-culture-as-key-causes-of-poverty/. Accessed 6 July 2018.

Schultz, Z. (2009). Update: Columbus teen dies after "Choking Game." WMTV-15 Madison, WI. http://www.nbc15.com/home/headlines/50646502.html. Accessed 6 July 2018.

Search Institute. (1997). https://www.search-institute.org/our-research/development-assets/. Accessed 6 July 2018.

SLJ. (2011). U.S. students rank 32 in math proficiency, 17 in reading, study says. *School Library Journal*. August 23, 2011. https://www.slj.com/2011/08/students/u-s-students-rank-32-in-math-proficiency-17-in-reading-study-says/#_. Accessed 6 July 2018.

Suttenfield, K. (2001). Report of the surgeon general's conference on children's mental health: A national action agenda. *Mental Health eJournal, 6*(1). https://www.medscape.com/viewarticle/430538. Accessed 6 July 2018.

Thakrar, A. P., Forrest, A. D., Maltenfort, M., & Forrest, C. B. (2018). Child mortality in the US and 19 OECD comparator nations: A 50-year time-trend analysis. *Health Affairs, 37*(1), 140–149. https://doi.org/10.1377/hlthaff.2017.0767.

Vitanna Organization. (n.d.). Teen pregnancy and poverty. https://vittana.org/teen-pregnancy-and-poverty. Accessed 6 July 2018.

Watts, L. (2011, February 28). Number of "dropout factories" declines. *Johns Hopkins Magazine*. http://archive.magazine.jhu.edu/2011/02/number-of-%E2%80%9Cdropout-factories%E2%80%9D-declines/. Accessed 6 July 2018.

Weinstock, H., et al. (2004). Sexually transmitted diseases among American youth. *Perspectives on Sexual & Reproductive Health, 36*, 6–10.

Weissbourd, R. (1997). *The vulnerable child: What really hurts America's children and what we can do about it.* New York: Da Capo Lifelong Books.

WHO. (2001). Mental health: A call for action by world health ministers. http://www.who.int/mental_health/advocacy/en/Call_for_Action_MoH_Intro.pdf. Accessed 6 July 2018.

Chapter 3
Child Abuse and Neglect in the United States

Abusive parents have inappropriate expectations of their children, with a reversal of dependence needs. Parents treat an abused child as if the child were older than the parents. A parent often turns to the child for reassurance, nurturing, comfort, and protection and expects a loving response.

Benjamin James Saddock, M.D.

All 50 states, the District of Columbia, and the US territories have child abuse and neglect reporting laws that mandate certain professionals and institutions to refer suspected maltreatment to a child protective services agency.

Each state has its own definition of child abuse and neglect that is based on standards set by federal law that identify a set of acts or behaviors that define child abuse and neglect. The Child Abuse Prevention and Treatment Act (CAPTA), as amended by the CAPTA Reauthorization Act of 2010, defines child abuse and neglect as any recent act or failure to act on the part of a parent or caretaker which results in death, serious physical or emotional harm, sexual abuse, and exploitation or an act or failure to act that presents an imminent risk of serious harm.

Most states recognize four major types of maltreatment: neglect, physical abuse, psychological maltreatment, and sexual abuse. Although any of the forms of child maltreatment occur separately, they can occur in combination as well.

The 2015 National Survey of Children's Exposure to Violence by the Office of Juvenile Justice and Delinquency Prevention reported that 57.7% of children in the United States experienced at least one exposure to (1) physical assault, (2) sexual victimization, (3) maltreatment, (4) property destruction, or (5) witnessing violence (OJJDP n.d). Among the individual categories of exposure, declines since 2008 outnumbered increases in 6 of the 54 types of exposure to violence covered in the survey.

States provide data for an annual Child Maltreatment report through the National Child Abuse and Neglect Data System (NCANDS), which was established in 1988 as a voluntary national data collection and analysis program to publish state child abuse and neglect information. Data has been collected every

© Springer Nature Switzerland AG 2019
J. C. Westman, *Dealing with Child Abuse and Neglect as Public Health Problems*, https://doi.org/10.1007/978-3-030-05897-5_3

year since 1991, and NCANDS now annually collects maltreatment data from child protective services agencies in the 50 states, the District of Columbia and the Commonwealth of Puerto Rico. Key findings in the 2018 NCANDS report include an increase from Fiscal Year 2015 to 2016 in three key metrics: referrals to child protective services (CPS) agencies alleging maltreatment (3.6%), referrals to CPS agencies accepted for investigation or alternative response (4.0%), and the number of children who were the subject of an investigation or alternative response (3.3%). Of the 3.5 million children who were the subject of an investigation or alternative response in Fiscal Year 2016, a national estimate of 676,000 children were victims of abuse and neglect, representing a 1.0% decrease from Fiscal Year 2015. In total, 74.8% of victims suffered neglect either by itself or in combination with any maltreatment type.

The national estimate of children who received a child protective services investigation response or alternative response increased 9% from 2011 to 2015. 75.3% of the victims were neglected, 17.2% were physically abused, and 8.4% were sexually abused. Children in their 1st year of life had the highest rate of victimization at 24.2 per 1000 children of the same age in the national population. A child may have suffered from multiple forms of maltreatment. The victims' ethnicities were 43.2% White, 23.6% Hispanic, 21.4% Black, and 11.8% others.

Juvenile ageism actually was identified early in the last century. Maria Montessori called attention to the "universal prejudices" against children, particularly in the attitude that adults always know what is best for them (Montessori 1969).

Child abuse and neglect result in physical and mental health damage. In addition, child abuse can leave epigenetic marks on a child's genes. Although they do not cause mutations in the DNA itself, the chemical modifications—including DNA methylation—change gene expression by silencing (or activating) genes. This can alter fundamental biological processes and adversely affect health outcomes throughout life (Mehta et al. 2013).

3.1 Who Reports Child Maltreatment?

In 2015, professionals made 63.4% of the reports alleging child abuse and neglect. The term professional means that the person had contact with the alleged child maltreatment victim as part of her or his job. This includes teachers, police officers, lawyers, and social services staff. The highest percentages of reports came from education personnel (18.4%), legal and law enforcement personnel (18.2%), and social services personnel (10.9%). Nonprofessionals—including friends, neighbors, and relatives—submitted 18.2% of the reports. Unclassified sources submitted the remainder.

3.2   How Many Children Die from Abuse or Neglect?

In 2015, an estimated 1670 children died of abuse and/or neglect at a rate of 2.25 per 100,000 children in the national population, according to data from the NCANDS. This is 5.7% more than in 2011 and translates into an average of nearly five children dying every day from abuse and/or neglect. NCANDS defines "child fatality" as the death of a child caused by an injury resulting from abuse or neglect or where abuse or neglect was a contributing factor.

Fatal child abuse may involve repeated abuse over a period of time, or it may involve a single, impulsive incident (e.g., drowning, suffocating, or shaking a baby). In cases of fatal neglect, the child's death results not from anything the caregiver does but from a caregiver's failure to act. The neglect may be chronic, e.g., extended malnourishment, or acute, e.g., a baby who drowns after being left unsupervised in a bathtub. In 2015, 72.9% of children who died from child maltreatment suffered neglect either alone or in combination with another maltreatment type, and 43.9% suffered physical abuse either alone or in combination with other maltreatment. Medical neglect either alone or in combination with another maltreatment type was reported in 7.3% of fatalities.

Boys had a higher child fatality rate than girls at 2.42/100,000 boys in the population and 2.09/100,000 girls. Of child fatalities, 42.3% were White, 30.6% were Black, 14.5% were Hispanic, and 12.6% were of other races.

The Centers for Disease Control and Prevention researchers found that persons who experienced considerable trauma during childhood died 20 years prematurely (Stevens 2009).

3.3   Who Are the Abusers and the Neglectful?

A perpetrator is the person who is responsible for the abuse or neglect of a child. According to the Children's Bureau report Child Maltreatment 2015, 522,476 perpetrators were reported in the United States. According to the analyses performed on the perpetrators (HHS 2015):

- 83.4% of perpetrators were between the ages of 18 and 44 years.
- 54.1% of perpetrators were women, 45% were men, and 0.9% were of unknown gender.
- 48.7% of perpetrators were White, 20% were Black, 19.5% Hispanic, and 11.8% other ethnicities.
- 61.5% of perpetrators maltreated one victim, 21.5% maltreated two victims, and the remaining 17% maltreated three or more victims.

3.4   Our Violent Society

Half of the children in the United States have been exposed to violence either as victims or as witnesses. Nearly five children die every day from either neglect or abuse or both. These facts are not openly recognized nor publicized. The widespread sexual abuse of children also calls out for public attention.

In addition to abuse and neglect, there often are environmental stresses in the form of neighborhood violence, economic hardship, substance abuse, or conflict between family members. Studies need to focus on both sources of stress in order to fully assess their impact on individual children (Sousa et al. 2018).

References

HHS [U.S. Department of Health and Human Services]. (2015). *Child maltreatment 2015*. https://www.acf.hhs.gov/sites/default/files/cb/cm2015.pdf. Accessed 6 July 2018.

Mehta, D., Klengel, T., et al. (2013). Childhood maltreatment is associated with distinct genomic and epigenetic profiles in posttraumatic stress disorder. *Proceedings of the National Academy of Sciences, 110*(20), 8302–8307. http://www.pnas.org/content/110/20/8302. Accessed 6 July 2018.

Montessori, M. (1969). *The formation of man* (trans: Joosten, A.M.) (p. 99). Madras: Theosophical Publishing House.

OJJDP [Office of Juvenile Justice and Delinquency Prevention]. (n.d.). National survey of children's exposure to violence. https://www.ojjdp.gov/research/national-survey-of-childrens-exposure-to-violence.html. Accessed 6 July 2018.

Sousa, C., Mason, W., et al. (2018). Direct and indirect effects of child abuse and environmental stress: A life-course perspective on adversity and depressive symptoms. *American Journal of Orthopsychiatry, 88*(2), 180–188.

Stevens, J. (2009). Traumatic childhood takes 20 years off life expectancy. *LJ World*. http://www2.ljworld.com/news/2009/oct/06/traumatic-childhood-takes-20-years-life-expectancy/. Accessed 6 July 2018.

Chapter 4
Child Sexual Abuse

> *In order to escape accountability for his crimes, the perpetrator does everything in his power to promote forgetting. If secrecy fails, the perpetrator attacks the credibility of his victim. If he cannot silence her absolutely, he tries to make sure no one listens.*
>
> Judith Lewis Herman (2015)

Research conducted by the Centers for Disease Control and Prevention estimates that approximately one in six boys and one in four girls are sexually abused before the age of 18 (USDOJ n.d.).

The tendency of victims to remain silent about rape and incest protects abusers. The abuse might involve varying degrees of pleasure and guilt that complicate the responses of victims. At the same time, some adolescents falsely allege abuse when parents frustrate their wishes. Still, even these allegations are cries for help for the family.

A meta-analysis of North American studies by Rebecca Bolen and Maria Scannapieco published in *Social Service Review* revealed that men and women who experienced childhood sexual abuse attempt suicide at twice the rate of those reporting no sexual abuse, have a 40% increased risk of marrying an alcoholic, and are at a 45% increased risk of marital problems (Bolen and Scannapieco 1999; USDOJ n.d.). Additional outcomes include substance abuse, running away from home, early menarche, and early pregnancy.

Child sexual abuse includes a wide range of sexual behaviors that take place between a child and an older person. These behaviors are meant to arouse the older person in a sexual way. In general, no thought is given to the effect the behavior may have on the child. For the most part, abusers are preoccupied with their own feelings and impulses and do not care about the reactions of the children.

Child sexual abuse often involves body contact. This could include sexual kissing; touching; and oral, anal, or vaginal sex. Not all sexual abuse involves body contact. Showing private parts ("flashing"), forcing children to watch pornography,

© Springer Nature Switzerland AG 2019
J. C. Westman, *Dealing with Child Abuse and Neglect as Public Health Problems*, https://doi.org/10.1007/978-3-030-05897-5_4

verbal pressure for sex, and exploiting children as prostitutes or for pornography can be sexual abuse as well.

Statutory rape occurs when an older person sexually penetrates a minor or a mentally handicapped person who, under state law, is incapable of consenting to sex. These persons deserve special protection because of their vulnerability. A person may be convicted of statutory rape even the victim explicitly consented and no force was used. Furthermore, a defendant may not use being mistaken about the person's age or incapacity as a defense. Most rape statutes specify that rape occurs when the victim is under a certain age and the perpetrator is over a certain age. For example, in Minnesota, criminal sexual conduct in the first degree is defined as sexual contact with a person under 13 years of age by a person who is more than 36 months older than the victim (Minnesota Statutes 2017).

4.1   Who Commits Child Sexual Abuse?

- Most often, sexual abusers know the children they abuse, but are not family members. For example, the abuser might be a friend of the family, babysitter, teacher, or neighbor. About six out of ten abusers fall into this group.
- About three out of ten of those who sexually abuse children are family members of the child. This includes fathers, uncles, or cousins.
- The abuser is a stranger in only about one out of ten child sexual abuse cases.
- Abusers are men in most cases, whether the victim is a boy or a girl.
- Women are the abusers in about 14% of cases reported against boys and about 6% of cases reported against girls.
- Child pornographers and other abusers who are strangers may make contact with children using the Internet.

4.2   What Are the Effects of Childhood Sexual Abuse?

It is not always easy to tell whether a child has been sexually abused. Sexual abuse often occurs in secret, and there is no physical proof of the abuse. For these reasons, child sexual abuse can be hard to detect.

Some child sexual abuse survivors may show symptoms of PTSD with anxiety, bad dreams, and other fears and worries. They may act out aspects of the abuse in their play. Young children may lose skills they once learned and act younger than they are. For example, an abused child might start wetting the bed or sucking her or his thumb. Some sexual abuse survivors show out-of-place sexual behaviors that are not expected in a child. They may act seductively or may not maintain safe limits with others. Children, especially boys, might "act out" with behavior problems. This could include being cruel to others and running away. Other children "act in" by becoming depressed. They may withdraw from friends or family. Older children or teens might try to hurt or even kill themselves.

Sexual abuse can be very confusing for children because it often involves being used or hurt by a trusted adult. The child might learn that the only way to get attention or love is to give something sexual or give up their self-respect. Some children believe the abuse is somehow their fault. They may think the abuser chose them because they must have wanted it or because there is something wrong with them. If the abuser was of the same sex, children (and parents) might wonder if that means they are gay.

Almost every child sexual abuse victim describes the abuse as negative. Most children know it is wrong. They usually have feelings of fear, shock, anger, and disgust. A small number of abused children might not realize it is wrong if they are very young or have developmental delays. Also, some victims might enjoy the attention, closeness, and physical contact with the abuser. This is more likely if these basic needs are not met by their caregivers. All told, these reactions make the abuse very difficult and confusing for children.

If childhood sexual abuse is not treated, long-term symptoms can continue through adulthood. These may include:

- PTSD and anxiety
- Depression and thoughts of suicide
- Sexual anxiety and disorders, including having too many or unsafe sexual partners
- Difficulty setting safe limits with others (e.g., saying no to others) and relationship problems
- Poor body image and low self-esteem
- Unhealthy behaviors, such as alcohol, drug, self-harm, or eating problems

These behaviors often are used to try to hide painful emotions related to the abuse. Anyone who was sexually abused as a child and has any of these symptoms should obtain professional help.

4.3   What Can Caregivers Do to Help Keep Children Safe?

Although caregivers cannot protect their children all of the time, it is important for them to know the people who have contact with their children. They can find out whether someone has been charged with sexual abuse and find out where sexual abusers live in their area by going to the website FamilyWatchdog.com. Most importantly, they need to provide a safe, caring environment so that their children feel able to talk to them about sexual abuse. Other tips to keep children safe include:

- Talk to others who know the people with whom your child comes in contact.
- Talk to your children about the difference between safe touching and unsafe touching.

- Tell your children that if someone tries to touch their body in their private areas or do things that make the child feel unsafe, they should say no to that person and tell you about it right away.
- Let children know that their bodies are private and that they have the right not to allow others to touch their bodies in any awkward way.
- Let them know that they do not have to do everything a babysitter, family member, or group leader tells them to do.
- Tell your children that abusers may use the Internet and set parental controls.

4.4   What Should You Do if You Think Your Child Has Been Sexually Abused?

If your child says she or he has been abused, try to stay calm. Reassure him or her that what happened is not her or his fault and that you are proud of him or her for telling you (or another person) and that you are there to keep her or him safe. Take your child to a mental health and medical professional right away. Many cities have child advocacy centers where a child and her family can get help. These centers interview children and family members in a sensitive, warm place. They can help you report the abuse to legal authorities. They can help you find a medical examiner and therapist skilled in child sexual abuse. The National Children's Alliance website has more information and a listing of appropriate centers.

Children can recover from sexual abuse and go on to live good lives. The best predictor of recovery is support and love from their main caregivers. As a caregiver, you might also consider getting help for yourself. It is often very hard to accept that your child has been sexually abused. You will not be supporting your child, though, if you respond in certain unhelpful ways. For example, you will not be able to provide support if you are overwhelmed by your own emotions. Do not downplay the abuse ("it wasn't that bad"), but also try not to have extreme fears related to the abuse ("my child will never be safe again"). It will not help children if you force them to talk or if you blame them. Getting therapy for yourself can help you deal with your own feelings about the abuse. Then you might be better able to provide support to your child.

4.4.1   Recommended Books About Child Sexual Abuse

- *My Body Is Private* by Linda Walvoord Girard and Rodney Pate (1992)
- *Please Tell! A Child's Story About Sexual Abuse* by Jessie Ottenweller (1991)
- *Something Happened to Me* by Phyllis E. Sweet (1985)
- *It Happens to Boys Too* by Jane Satullo and Russell Bradway (1987)

- *The Courage to Heal: A Guide for Women Survivors of Child Sexual Abuse* (4th edition) by Ellen Bass and Laura Davis (2008)
- *Wounded Boys Heroic Men: A Man's Guide to Recovering from Child Abuse* by Daniel Jay Sonkin and Lenore E. A. Walker (1998)
- *Parenting Errors: How to Solve Them* by Kerby T. Alvy (2017)

4.5 Sexual Abuse and the Catholic Church

The Vatican has done much to address clergy members' sexual abuse of children, which has threatened to stain the entire church (Pope Benedict XVI once memorably called it "filth"). It has removed abusive priests, worked more closely with local law enforcement officials, toughened its regulations and generally adopted a "zero tolerance" approach.

The Vatican hosted a 4-day Congress "Child Dignity in the Digital World" in October, 2017, devoted to the spreading scourge of online child pornography. It was an opportunity to strike a positive note about the Vatican's role in protecting minors (Horowitz and Goodstein 2017). That Congress sought ways to protect children in what has been depicted as a frightening digital world, where abusers surf a dark web and child pornography proliferates. It included experts in the field speaking about the risks as more children in developing countries go online. They discussed troubling statistics, such as the finding last year by the Internet Watch Foundation, that more than 57,000 websites contained images of children being sexually abused. Catholic representatives have been on panels, such as the International Politics and Law Regarding Child Sexual Abuse.

But in an awkward confluence of events, the 2017 Vatican Congress took place mere weeks after the Holy See recalled Monsignor Carlo Capella, a church diplomat in the Vatican Embassy in Washington, amid accusations that he had possessed child pornography. The Canadian police had issued an arrest warrant for Monsignor Capella accusing him of distributing child pornography during a Christmas visit in 2016 to Ontario. This was another of the abuse accusations against priests that have dogged the church around the globe for decades even as it has promised to punish predators and protect the preyed upon.

Advocates for victims have argued that the Vatican's invocation of diplomatic immunity to recall Monsignor Capella from the United States shows that it still prioritizes protecting its own. They say they consider the Capella case a shameful echo of an earlier episode involving Jozef Wesolowski, a Polish archbishop accused of abusing children in the Dominican Republic where he served as the Vatican ambassador (Goodstein 2014). The Vatican removed the archbishop and denied appeals that he be tried in the Dominican Republic. He was defrocked and died in the Vatican before facing justice.

In his speech before top Italian officials and representatives from Interpol, the United Nations, Russia, China, the United States, Facebook, and Microsoft, Cardinal Parolin spoke at length about the growing threat of Internet abuse on the spirit and psyches of young users. He acknowledged that when it came to the exploitation and abuse of children, "over the past few decades, this tragic reality has come powerfully to the fore in the Catholic Church, and extremely grave facts have emerged."

But critics say Vatican action has lagged behind the Vatican's words. For example, a tribunal to discipline bishops who cover up abuse was disbanded because, the Pope said, the Vatican already had the requisite offices to deal with the issue. A commission Pope Francis created with top cardinals, outside experts, and abuse victims (the committee's only two victims have since left) has seemed to be stifled by Vatican bureaucracy. In addition, the Pope brought Cardinal George Pell to Rome as a senior despite allegations of abuse against him. Cardinal Pell is now back in Australia facing charges of sexual assault against minors. Rev. Hans Zollner, a member of the Pontifical Commission for the Protection of Minors, said he was confident that this time, the accused cleric would face justice. "Everyone who commits a crime needs to be punished," he said. "Period."

For years, top Vatican officials in Rome had dismissed the abuse crisis as a unique product of the Anglo-Saxon world and suggested that it had been overplayed by the news media. But organizers of the 2017 Vatican Congress said the majority of the experts came from countries in the global North because that is where the problem has been confronted most aggressively.

In an interview, Father Zollner said that on his global travels looking into the problem, he had observed that bishops and clerics in countries such as Malawi were finally facing an issue they would not talk about as recently as a year ago. But other nations still are constrained by local cultural taboos about discussing child abuse, he said. Italy, he noted, was not without its own bombshell reports of sexual abuse in the church. He compared the book *Lust* about abuse in the Vatican by the investigative journalist Emiliano Fittipaldi to the breakthrough reports by The Boston Globe's Spotlight team on the cover-up of priests' sexual abuse of children (O'Connell 2017). Father Zollner said the media focus on Monsignor Capella could have a positive side effect and put "more attention to the topic of the Vatican Congress," which, he said, was to better understand the phenomenon of child pornography and how to prevent it. "That is our whole purpose," he said.

On January 16, 2018, Pope Francis said that he was "pained and ashamed" over the "irreparable damage" priests had inflicted on minors (Londono 2018). This has contributed to the loss of millions of followers of the Catholic Church in Latin America. Between 1995 and 2017, the number of Chileans who described themselves as Catholic dropped from 74% to 45%, according to a poll conducted by Latinobarómetro.

4.6   Our Sexually Abusive Society

The estimate that one in six boys and one in four girls have been sexually abused before the age of 18 in the United States adds sexual abuse to violence as a social problem that must be addressed.

The Catholic Church is in a position to pursue advocacy for children because of its awareness of their vulnerability to sexual abuse and its devotion to serving their interests.

Significantly, the sexual abuse of adult women has gained national attention and action plans because of their ability to make public disclosures of their abuse. This is unlikely to happen for children because they are not able to do so and because of power of juvenile ageism.

References

Bolen, R. M., & Scannapieco, M. (1999). Prevalence of child sexual abuse: A corrective meta-analysis. *Social Service Review, 73*(3), 281–313.

Goodstein, L. (2014). For Nuncio accused of abuse, dominicans want justice at home, not abroad. *The New York Times*. https://www.nytimes.com/2014/08/24/world/americas/whisked-away-vatican-ambassador-accused-of-sexual-abuse-of-minors.html. Accessed 6 July 2018.

Herman, J. L. (2015). *Trauma and recovery: The aftermath of violence – from domestic abuse to political terror* (1st revised ed.). New York: Basic Books.

Horowitz, J. & Goodstein, L. (2017). Vatican sex abuse scandal reveals blind spot for Francis. *The New York Times*. https://www.nytimes.com/2017/06/29/world/europe/cardinal-pell-charges-australia.html?_r=0. Accessed 6 July 2018.

Londono, E. (2018). In Chile, Pope apologizes for "Damage" from abuse. *The New York Times,* p. A4. https://www.nytimes.com/2018/01/16/world/americas/pope-francis-chile-sexual-abuse.html. Accessed 6 July 2018.

Minnesota Statutes Ann. (2017). § 609.342 [West 1996]. https://www.revisor.mn.gov/statutes/?id=609.342. Accessed 6 July 2018.

O'Connell, G. (2017). New book by Vatileaks journalist alleges Vatican inaction on sexual abuse. *America – The Jesuit Review*. https://www.americamagazine.org/faith/2017/01/19/new-book-vatileaks-journalist-alleges-vatican-inaction-sexual-abuse. Accessed 6 July 2018.

USDOJ [U.S. Department of Justice]. (n.d.). Raising awareness about sexual abuse. *Facts and Statistics*. https://www.nsopw.gov/en-US/Education/FactsStatistics. Accessed 6 July 2018.

Chapter 5
Juvenile Ageism

> Youth is a wonderful thing.
> What a crime to waste it on children!
>
> George Bernard Shaw

George Bernard Shaw opened the door to understanding where young people really stand in our society. Even children might smile at Shaw's cynical humor. However, if the words Jews, Blacks, or gays are substituted for children, prejudice is instantly apparent. The fact that we do not take offense at this slur against children illustrates how ingrained our hidden prejudice is against them.

When I point this out, you still will likely doubt the existence of juvenile ageism. After all, we are just referring to children, and they are not protesting…or so it seems. More to the point, why should anyone suggest prejudice and discrimination when children receive so much media attention and often are overindulged at home? They are better off now than a century ago because we protect them with child labor and abuse and neglect laws. We spend billions on public education and on supporting teen parents.

But a different picture emerges if we heed the National Commission on Children. It concluded over 20 years ago that our nation was failing its children (Kortet Task Force 2003). The fact that we are still failing them is reflected in the violence, habitual crime, and welfare dependency that plague our society today and the evidence presented in Chap. 1. Our children are protesting the consequences of juvenile ageism indeed.

Many people are weary of the claims of victims of racism, sexism, classism, and elder ageism. They understandably feel that we do not need another -ism. They correctly believe that prejudice and discrimination always have been and always will be a part of the human condition. But public consciousness of racism, sexism, and elder ageism has led to counteractive attitudes and actions.

We need to think objectively about juvenile ageism as a destructive force. The history of the gradual evolution of actions to counteract racism, sexism, and elder ageism helps answer why awareness of juvenile ageism is essential for our society's well-being and can be activated.

© Springer Nature Switzerland AG 2019

J. C. Westman, *Dealing with Child Abuse and Neglect as Public Health Problems*, https://doi.org/10.1007/978-3-030-05897-5_5

5.1   Historic Prejudices

There was a time when the exploitation of Blacks in the United States was justified by the belief that they were naturally inferior and destined to servitude and ignorance. They were regarded as either a different kind of being or at an earlier stage of evolution than Caucasians. They had inferior emotional control and moral capacities like children. Education was wasted on them because they were incapable of learning. A male adult was called "boy" with all that word's negative implications. He was regarded as a child who needed guidance and direction.

Institutional racism in the South continued after the Civil War. It shifted from benevolent to malevolent forms as Blacks were lynched, and Whites avoided prosecution for crimes against them. Their inferior education, medical care, jobs, housing, representation, and legal services are documented in an extensive literature.

Largely due to the Civil Rights Movement of the 1950s and 1960s, Blacks developed a positive group identity, and overt discrimination was outlawed. Although racism remains an important issue, substantial progress has been made to overcome it.

Women have been presumed to be weak, emotional, lacking ambition, illogical, and unfit for managerial or technical jobs. They have been considered as dependent as are children. Stereotypes denied women the educational and career opportunities available to men. To this day, the results are less pay for the same work and a glass ceiling that can limit workplace promotions.

Waves of feminist movements over the years culminated in equal rights legislation. Marriage is now characterized as a relationship between two individuals with equal personal rights. But just as Blacks have shown prejudice against other Blacks, women have shown prejudice against other women. This is most visible when discussing the priority given to homemaking and childrearing versus paid careers.

The public's awareness of sexism has extended beyond a single gender as prejudice and discrimination against males have begun to gain recognition, such as with boys in some female-dominated classrooms.

Classism is prejudice and discrimination based on different social or economic groups. The family into which a person is born determines that person's place in society. The traditional example is India's caste system. Still, an American birth family shapes every person's life almost as surely.

The Horatio Alger theme claims that anyone can achieve anything in America, so the existence of classism is usually denied. The predominant view of the United States is that of a classless meritocracy and a land of unbounded opportunity. The theme that anyone can become president was reinforced by the election of Barack Obama (2006) who wrote *Dreams from My Father: A Story of Race and Inheritance* as described in the following review:

> A brilliant but troubled Kenyan father abandoned his teenage bride and their infant son. Obama described a footloose mother who took "Barry" to Indonesia with a second husband, then shipped him back to Hawaii to live with his grandparents. He felt a sense of alienation as a young black man growing up with few Black friends or role models. Chubby

as a kid, wayward as a teen, he developed formidable personal discipline, down to his daily exercise routine and abstemious eating and drinking habits. He made a home for himself in Chicago and sought out the stability of marriage and fatherhood. He successfully pursued a career in politics.

Nevertheless, social class strongly influences destiny. Chuck Collins and Felice Yeskel (2005) demonstrate this in their book *Economic Apartheid in America*. Contrary to popular belief, our nation was not established as a true democracy. Only White men who owned property initially had the right to vote.

Wealthy people always have enjoyed advantages over working class people. A popular myth is that the wealthy earn their fortunes through hard work and effort. Average Americans work very hard indeed, yet when adjusted for inflation, their wages have been in serious decline for years even as their productivity has increased. Workers are producing more and earning less. Meanwhile, corporate profits and CEO salaries based on corporate revenues have increased.

Classism occurs in both downward and upward directions. This is especially evident during political campaigns that exaggerate populism and elitism. Poor mothers are portrayed as "welfare queens," university professors are "out of touch with reality," and the wealthy are "conscienceless, money-grubbing pirates" who exploit the middle class.

5.2 Ageism

In 1969, the physician Robert Butler described ageism as prejudice and institutional discrimination against the elderly in housing, employment, and health care (Achenbaum 2015). More specifically, gerontophobia—fear of aging—was identified as a prejudice that led to discrimination by avoiding the elderly and by elder abuse. In 1970, the Gray Panthers was created as an advocacy group to combat ageism. The following year, President Nixon condemned ageism in his address to the White House Conference on Aging.

The Group for the Advancement of Psychiatry identified ageism as avoidance of elders by younger individuals. This particular form of discrimination was created by a society "that regards death as a personal affront and that values the action, vigor, and skills of youth over the contemplation, experience and wisdom of old age."

The elderly are presumed to be inferior in physical strength, in mental abilities, and in their awareness of the surrounding world. They are considered dependent on others, like children, due to the physical and mental decline that accompanies aging. Intriguingly, elder abuse and neglect have been readily identified as reflecting ageism, whereas childhood abuse and neglect have not. Of course, older persons are politically organized to protect their interests and claim abuse, while the young are unrepresented and unable to protect their own interests.

Since the young and the old are both dependent on society, they actually have much in common. They are both financially dependent because they do not earn income. This can place the duty and the burden for their support on their families and government. They compete against each other for government funds. Unless elders are motivated by a sense of responsibility for the young and the future, their political power easily overwhelms the interests of the young and planning for our society's economic future. The duty of all adults to provide for the next generation is easily neglected in our political systems.

Sacrificing for our children's present and future well-being has inherent moral attraction. Thus, no platitude is more frequently invoked and more frequently disregarded when it comes time for action than "Do it for our kids."

The young have seldom been included in descriptions of ageism; even when they are, the references have been limited to young adults. Ironically, the educational literature for children refers to ageism only as it affects the elderly. In fact, psychologist Todd Nelson's (2002) book *Ageism* defines ageism exclusively as prejudice and discrimination of the young against the elderly. This exclusion of children whose status is defined by age from ageism is the ultimate expression of juvenile ageism.

Juvenile ageism actually was identified early in the last century. Maria Montessori (1969) called attention to the "universal prejudices" against children, particularly in the attitude that adults always know what is best for them. She cited the false assumptions that children must be taught to learn, which overlooks their innate thirst for learning; that children's minds are empty, which overlooks their rich imaginations; and that young children do not work, which overlooks the growth-inducing nature of play.

Obvious signs of juvenile ageism can be seen today in public displays. The Child-Free Network is a support group for adults without children. *How to be a Happy Parent…in Spite of Your Children* is a book title that needs no further comment. A newspaper ad urged readers: "If you don't own a kid, borrow one and catch 'Great Big Tour' in the Oscar Mayer Theatre." In the play The Gingerbread House, the father says, "Honey, I think we should sell our kids. We can start our lives again."

Again, imagine your response if the word Jews, Blacks, or gays was substituted for kids.

5.3 Victimization of Young Persons

Prejudice occurs when judgments are made before facts are determined and weighed. It refers to any unreasonable attitude of superiority over others and often is triggered by competition for space, material things, or time.

Discrimination occurs when prejudiced people are given superior access to resources. Individuals are treated differently based on their group membership or category rather than on merit. Discrimination takes both individual and social forms. The first type consists of overt acts that harm others. The second type is more subtle and difficult to spot. This kind of covert discrimination operates within established and often respected influences in our society.

Discrimination is reinforced by the compliance of victims as well as their rebellious reactions. When victims lash out, they are blamed for the frustrations and guilt of the prejudiced. A clear-cut example is found with delinquent teenagers. They are victims of our society's failure to ensure that they have competent parents and safe neighborhoods. Their rebellious behavior is punished without addressing its obvious causes and our unrecognized guilt for ignoring their long-standing plight.

Victims of prejudice are treated differently because they are different in appearance, interests, and sophistication. Children's natural physical, mental, and resource inferiority makes them dependent on others and vulnerable to prejudice and discrimination. Their dependence along with their natural inclination to challenge authority makes them prime targets when they compete with adults for space, resources, emotional involvement, and time or when they make adults anxious.

Dependents of any age threaten our independence. They require personal sacrifices that change the status quo. The birth of a child alters a parent's life even more dramatically than an elderly parent's incapacity. Although affection for and commitment to a dependent person make those sacrifices possible, the inevitable result is personal loss, inconvenience, and some degree of resentment. In this context, a dependent person can be seen as inferior and less deserving than an independent adult. Dependent persons also are a burden for anyone who pays taxes.

Moreover, prejudice and discrimination can be expressed in benevolent and idealizing ways. For example, before racism was considered a social problem, many people believed slaves were content and needed direction. Before sexism was challenged, many people believed women were dependent and were satisfied with a subservient status. The idealization of motherhood continues to help men avoid childrearing tasks with their own children.

Benevolent prejudice underlies the pro-children rhetoric that allows adults to feel good. Thinking and speaking about our devotion to children helps to conceal discrimination against them. It enables a lack of action that might fulfill our responsibilities. Benevolent ageism also allows us to believe that the elderly are better off receiving special care away from their families and that children are better off in educational environments away from their families.

Many of us believe the material wishes of our children should be gratified or that our children should have better lives than we did. We do not recognize that overly protective and indulgent attitudes prevent our children from learning how to handle life's challenges and opportunities. Because children really are dependent, the guise of protecting and indulging them conceals juvenile ageism and their need to learn how to assume personal responsibility. The harmful effects are less evident because children's missed opportunities and challenges do not occur until far into the future.

Benevolent juvenile ageism can take other forms. When children are viewed as capable, rational, and independent in order to justify less parental involvement, they again become victims. Over the past 30 years, children's capabilities have increasingly been seen as better developed by professionals than by their parents. This creates jobs in childcare and early childhood education and frees parents for paid employment.

These children prematurely regarded as independent presumably can then achieve the American ideal of individual freedom. They quickly shed signs of their vulnerability, neediness, or bewilderment as they adopt the cool persona of the sophisticated children in commercialized images. A common example is the teenage gangs' hip-hop lifestyle, which nurtures nihilism, misogyny, and bravado and conceals insecurity and immaturity. All of this undermines childhood and adolescence as long, legitimate life stages during which our young prepare for fulfilling and responsible lives through cultural lessons provided by competent parents.

As long ago as the early 1980s, the writer Marie Winn (1984) in her book *Children without Childhood* called attention to children who grow up without experiencing childhood. Neil Postman (1994) reiterated this theme in his book *The Disappearance of Childhood*. The pressure placed on children to act like adults and its commercial exploitation is vividly illustrated by this 2011 anecdote from Newsweek:

> Five-year-old Olivia Myers is an indefatigable clothes horse. "She's had a great eye from a very early age," says her mother, Alyse. Take the flirty ensemble the youthful New Yorker angled off to school in last week. In low-slung, torso-tight flowered bell bottoms with a frothy white "poet" blouse from her favorite boutique, "Little Leepers," Olivia sashayed with the poise of any nubile Lolita bound for a discotheque—except she's about a third the size. "She's five and three quarters years old going on 15," says her mother proudly.

Premature introduction to sexual activity is an acknowledged example of the loss of childhood. One in five adolescents says they have electronically sent or posted online nude or seminude images of themselves. About 40% have had nude/seminude images originally meant to be private shared with them. An online survey by TRU indicates that more than a third say that exchanging sexy words and pictures makes "hooking up" with others more likely (National Campaign n.d.).

At the same time, Garrison Keillor noted that childhood and adolescence have been stolen by adults. Immaturity has become the norm rather than the exception. Men refuse to grow up; husbands in their 30s enjoy playing the same video games that obsess 12-year-olds; young men and women will not commit to marriage or family; and fathers fight with umpires or coaches at little league games. Keillor (1994) put it this way in *The Book of Guys*:

> Years ago, manhood was an opportunity for achievement, and now it is a problem to overcome...boy-men fixate on adolescent longings for the intensity and variety of experience and escape from their parents and family...over time they have abandoned traditional markers of male maturity and embraced perpetual adolescence. Commercial culture reinforces both trends.

Keillor's point is affirmed by Diana West (2007) in her book *The Death of the Grown-Up*.

Underlying the tendency to denigrate childhood is the disparagement of anyone who is small, weak, or needy. We prize size, strength, and self-sufficiency. As a result, childhood and adolescence tend to be regarded as necessary evils on the pathway to adulthood. They are to be passed through as quickly as possible rather than be experienced as legitimate phases of life to be lived fully.

5.4   Arguments Against the Existence of Juvenile Ageism

The argument can be made that whatever difficulties America's children have individually or collectively do not reflect prejudice or discrimination. Adversity is part of life. Children and adults can suffer because they are innocent bystanders, as happens in war. Children and adults can fall victim to misfortune, poverty, bad parenting, racism, and sexism. Child neglect and abuse can spring from parental deficiencies, illnesses, or disorders without prejudice or discrimination against the children.

The existence of juvenile ageism also can be dismissed on the grounds that parents represent the interests of their children. They may do so imperfectly but mistakes do not constitute prejudice or discrimination. The power adults have over children comes from their legal and socioeconomic privileges, greater resources, and nurturing capacities.

Moreover, the interests of adults without children are becoming increasingly dominant. The interests of children who presumably are significant only to their parents can be overridden by the will of the majority. A tangible by-product of this trend was the disappearance of the traditional family wage by the equalization of pay for adults with and without children.

A particular objection to juvenile ageism is that our democratic republic is based upon competing interests in our political system. Since children are not represented, their plight is not a reflection of prejudice or discrimination; it is simply the result of governments that only represent registered voters.

Another objection is that unsafe neighborhoods and violence result from poverty and racism; the fact that children are affected is incidental. That attitude might be valid in underdeveloped nations but is unjustifiable in a prosperous society. We cannot claim ignorance or lack of resources as excuses for leaving our children unprotected from poverty and violence. Since the cost is miniscule compared to wars, national security, and crime, we can easily access the resources to ensure their safety and competent parenting…if we have the will to do so.

5.5   Arguments for the Existence of Juvenile Ageism

In the distant past, fathers held life-and-death power over their children. Sons and daughters were regarded as property parents could treat as they wished. Over time, restrictions were placed on the rights of parents as societies became increasingly involved in the lives of children. Children have been accorded an increasing number of legal and civil rights over the last century.

The term adultism first appeared in psychological literature in 1933. It defined a child possessing the "physique and spirit" of an adult and who tended toward delinquency. In his seminal 1978 article "Adultism" in Adolescence, Jack Flasher redefined adultism as the belief that children are inferior (Flasher 1978; LeFrançois

2013). Adultism showed in excessive nurturing, possessiveness, or over-restrictiveness consciously or unconsciously designed to control a child.

Adultism was expanded by the Child Welfare League of America to include disempowering and disenfranchising youth by viewing them as objects instead of human beings (Delgado 2002). President Theodore Roosevelt recognized this injustice when he initiated a series of White House Conferences on Children and Youth held from 1909 to 1971.

Juvenile ageism is a more descriptive and understandable term than *adultism*, which can be construed to mean prejudice against adults, and than *childism*, which can imply childish behavior and omits adolescents. Juvenile ageism identifies age as the target and links the young with older people who also must contend with elder ageism.

Prejudice and discrimination against children were not described as juvenile ageism until the 1970s by Chester Pierce, a psychiatrist, and myself. In 1980, the pediatrician Michael Rothenberg suggested a hidden national conspiracy against children (Rothenberg 1980). As proof, he pointed out the vast discrepancy between pro-children rhetoric and the actions and inactions of our governments that expose the failure to implement that rhetoric.

How does juvenile ageism explain the variety of ways children are mistreated? When is maltreatment the result of juvenile ageism, and when is it the result of ignorance, incompetence, or just plain meanness? When the latter factors explain the maltreatment, does that automatically exclude juvenile ageism? Is a mentally ill parent who abuses a child a juvenile ageist? Is our society's inability to protect everyone from violence a sign of juvenile ageism when children become victims?

Answers to these questions can be found by comparing juvenile ageism with racism and sexism. Ask if all the abuse, neglect, and segregation of minorities and women can be blamed on racism and sexism. The answer clearly is no. Members of these groups can bring maltreatment upon themselves. They can be mistreated for reasons other than their race or gender.

We can identify the trends and instances that reflect the discriminatory practices of racism, sexism, and ageism by looking at the attitudes that motivate behavior. First, attitudes that reflect in-group superiority over an out-group, coupled with the power to dominate out-group members, signal an -ism. Second, -ism-based behavior exploits, maltreats or ignores people's needs because their personal characteristics differ from the dominant group. Those differences can be based on race, gender, class, or age.

In contrast, the maltreatment of others based on competition, conflicts of opinion or desires, envy or jealousy, and revenge need not reflect an -ism. This means that juvenile ageism exists when adults use their superior power to mistreat children as inferior persons in order to further their own needs and desires. By the same token, elders can be the victims of ageism when younger persons use their superior power to mistreat them to satisfy their own needs and desires.

Still, the idea of unequal treatment, which is central in racism and sexism, seems more complicated in juvenile ageism. Unlike racial and gender groups, children usually are inferior in mental and physical abilities. Children progress from complete dependency through obtaining increasing privileges and responsibilities. During that process, they require gradually diminishing supervision. Therefore, juvenile ageism cannot be invoked simply because children are treated differently due to their immaturity.

However, the comparison of elder and juvenile ageism with racism and sexism holds up when equality means equality in rights and opportunities. Ageists claim that the rights and opportunities of elders and children are less important than those of the majority of adults. Children, therefore, can be treated unequally, and their right to developmental opportunities can go unfulfilled. Elders also can be treated unequally, and opportunities to meet their rights and needs can be ignored or denied.

Specific psychological factors foster ageism. Adults are naturally ambivalent toward the elderly and the young because both restrict their independence. The elderly remind us that we will age and die. The young remind us of our childlike, dependent tendencies. These directly conflict with the priority we place on being independent and carefree. To ward off those anxieties, we might avoid the elderly and expect our children to be independent.

At a deeper level, those of us who are parents naturally hold some buried resentment toward our children because they require sacrifices. This resentment is accentuated by the competition between careers and childrearing demands. Moreover, many of us harbor shards of the frightened, hurt, or angry children we once were. This blocks true empathy with our children and creates either excessive anger or overprotection.

Most importantly, the premise held by adults without offspring that parents do not merit special consideration solely due to childrearing responsibilities denies the principle that all adults have a responsibility to support the continuation of our society through the next generation…posterity in the Declaration of Independence. It ignores the stake all adults have in preventing the costly products of struggling families: the Cradle to Prison/Welfare Dependency Pipeline.

5.6   Our Juvenile Ageist Society

Juvenile ageism is concealed by rhetoric that idealizes children even as we ignore their interests in adult affairs and their stake in our future economy. Our nation's failure to plan for the future of our children is not considered the same kind of failure as parents' failure to plan for their daughters' and sons' futures. Because the prejudice and discrimination of juvenile ageism is not recognized, we need to know more about these powerful hidden forces that victimize our young citizens.

References

Achenbaum, W. A. (2015). A history of ageism Since 1969. *Generations, Journal of the American Society on Aging.* http://www.asaging.org/blog/history-ageism-1969.

Collins, C., & Yeskel, F. (2005). *Economic apartheid in America: A primer on economic inequality & insecurity.* New York: The New Press.

Delgado, M. (2002). *New frontiers for youth development in the twenty-first century: Revitalizing and broadening youth development.* New York: Columbia University Press. https://epdf.tips/new-frontiers-for-youth-development-in-the-twenty-first-century.html. Accessed 6 July 2018.

Flasher, J. (1978). Adultism. *Adolescence, 13*(51), 517–523.

Keillor, G. (1994). *The book of guys.* New York: Penguin.

Kortet Task Force on K-12 Education. (2003). Are we still at risk? *Education Next, 3*(2). http://educationnext.org/are-we-still-at-risk/. Accessed 6 July 2018.

LeFrançois, B. (2013). Adultism. https://doi.org/10.1007/978-1-4614-5583-7_6. https://www.researchgate.net/publication/280102266_Adultism. Accessed 6 July 2018.

Montessori, M. (1969). *The formation of man* (p. 99) (trans: Joosten, A. M.). Madras: Theosophical Publishing House.

National Campaign to Prevent Teen and Unplanned Pregnancy. (n.d.). Sex and tech. https://www.drvc.org/pdf/protecting_children/sextech_summary.pdf. Accessed 6 July 2018.

Nelson, T. (Ed.). (2002). *Ageism: Stereotyping and prejudice against older persons.* Cambridge, MA: MIT Press.

Obama, B. (2006). *Dreams from my father: A story of race and inheritance.* New York: Crown Publishing Group.

Postman, N. (1994). *The disappearance of childhood.* New York: Vintage.

Rothenberg, M. B. (1980). Is there an unconscious national conspiracy against children in the United States? *Clinical Pediatrics, 19*(1), 10. 15–6, 21–4.

West, D. (2007). *The death of the grown-up: How America's arrested development is bringing down western civilization.* New York: St. Martin's Press.

Winn, M. (1984). *Children without childhoods: Growing up to fast in a world of sex and drugs.* New York: Penguin.

Chapter 6
Dynamics of Juvenile Ageism

The prejudice and discrimination of both elder and juvenile ageism can be identified in how power is wielded over rights and opportunities in relationship to age. The triad of (1) exploitation that uses, (2) maltreatment that demeans, and (3) neglect that ignores dependency is a form of discrimination that reflects an attitude of superiority.

6.1 Exploitation That Uses

Juvenile ageism serves a variety of purposes. On the positive side, children can enhance a parent's self-esteem when they respect and need their parents. On the negative side, children can be exploited when having one is used to build self-esteem and when children are seen as sources of affection, such as when girls seek to become pregnant. Whenever they are used primarily to satisfy their parents' needs, children are exploited through their parents' superior power.

Parents exploit children when they project unacceptable parts of themselves onto their children. In this way, we avoid painful feelings about ourselves. This is frequently seen in the physical abuse of children perceived as threatening. Another form of exploitation is to take out resentments and hostility toward another adult, often the other parent, on a helpless child.

Children can be exploited by being expected to fulfill their parents' expectations rather than their own potential. Steven graphically illustrated this theme:

Twenty-four-year-old Mary came to our clinic because eight-year-old Steven was unmanageable at home and at school. She was at her wits end and wanted "something done about Steven."

Mary was raised in an abusive home as the oldest of five children. Because of her parents' alcoholism and unpredictability, she raised her younger siblings. In the eyes of her mother she could "never do anything right." Her father hit her during alcohol-induced rages. She managed to get by in school and parent her siblings when her mother was

© Springer Nature Switzerland AG 2019
J. C. Westman, *Dealing with Child Abuse and Neglect as Public Health Problems*, https://doi.org/10.1007/978-3-030-05897-5_6

intoxicated. When she was sixteen, she deliberately became pregnant in order to get away from home. Her marriage ended in the first year because of her husband's irresponsibility and abuse. A series of relationships with unstable males followed, each one ending because they exploited her.

In family therapy, Mary revealed with a flood of tears her frightening insight that she had been taking out her longstanding resentment against males who exploited her on Steven. She could see that she was prejudiced against Steven and had been discriminating against him. Steven was transfixed when he observed his mother's emotions. He hadn't seen her cry this way before. He went to her and put his arms around her. They both cried together. With this reframing of the relationship between mother and son, Mary no longer needed to be a perpetrator. Steven no longer had to rebel as the victim of her prejudice and discrimination.

Mary and Steven are familiar to family therapists who commonly uncover scapegoating in families. The rebellion of the victim can be remedied by a more realistic and accepting attitude from the perpetrator. Understanding that you are prejudiced is the first step toward overcoming discrimination.

Many abusive parents were abused as children. When they abuse their sons and daughters, they are reacting to distorted views. They often expect their children to be "ideal parents" who give them love and respect. They feel betrayed when their children are just children who need guidance and make demands upon them.

Do distorted expectations mean that parental behavior is not prejudiced and discriminatory? This question can be answered by examining racism and sexism again. Certainly, many personal determinants exist in those -isms. Adults who have been discriminated against can be prejudiced themselves. In racism, darker-skinned Blacks can be prejudiced against people with lighter skin and vice versa. Insecure men dominate women. The essential question is whether abusive parents deny their children's rights and opportunities to serve their own needs. If the answer is yes, they are juvenile ageists.

Teachers, clergypersons, coaches, physicians, psychotherapists, and other adults in authority can abuse their power, especially when a child or adolescent offers affection or respect that is perceived as seductive. Under those circumstances, exploitative juvenile ageism occurs when the adult with superior power has an exploitative sexual relationship with a young person.

6.2 Maltreatment That Demeans

The most glaring forms of discrimination in juvenile ageism are violations of civil rights that would be regarded as rejection, segregation, harassment, oppression, violence, torture, and murder if they targeted an adult. Lumping together all these egregious offences under child abuse and neglect—less evocative terms—demeans children. Significantly, the death of a child from abuse often is not regarded as murder, and the word torture rarely is used to describe child abuse, even when children are chained in basements and beaten.

Most explanations for child neglect and abuse focus on socioeconomic and racial factors as if the quality of parenting played a minor role. Parental pathology, although recognized, is explained away as a reaction to stressful or disadvantaged circumstances. We especially demean children by solely blaming them rather than their parents when they become social problems and deal with them as if they were simply adult offenders.

Prejudice against children also is more subtly reflected in the demeaning attitude that children do not deserve more than their parents can provide. Inherent in this view is the belief that children are personal possessions of their parents without their own interests or rights. Children from disadvantaged families, therefore, do not deserve the same rights and opportunities as children from affluent families: "They don't deserve my support as a taxpayer. They aren't like me."

One of the reasons we do not act to prevent child neglect and abuse is that we are reluctant to judge parental competence. This gives parents an unchallenged superior position and enables them to exercise power over their children through neglect and abuse. By failing to prevent the familial and environmental factors associated with neglect and abuse by setting a standard for parenthood, we are withholding the power to protect (neglecting) children. It is an expression of juvenile ageism. Punishing children who are reacting to parental neglect and abuse is an even more clear-cut expression of juvenile ageism.

6.3   Neglect That Ignores Dependency

Is juvenile ageism really expressed when our society fails to protect our children from parental neglect and abuse? Here again the answer lies in our attitude. Do we regard our children as human beings with rights or as the personal property of their parents? Does ignoring incompetent parents before their children are damaged by abuse and/or neglect reflect a hidden dehumanizing attitude of adult superiority when we fail to exercise our power to protect our nation's children before they are damaged by neglect and or abuse? It does.

Protests against animal abuse are easily organized but have you ever heard of an organized protest against child abuse? We could explain that absence because animals are helpless and need protection. We could claim we do not know what to do about child abuse. We could say that childrearing is a totally private matter with no consequences for society. We could say that child neglect and abuse are not related to our society's violence, habitual crime, and welfare dependency. But we know that none of these statements are true.

Incompetent parents obviously neglect and abuse children. Yet, we do not recognize incompetent parenting as a public health and national economic risk even though it is more important than environmental toxins, poverty, malnutrition, and missed immunizations. If we seriously want to prevent child neglect and abuse, we need to acknowledge (1) that we do know about the problem, (2) that we do know what to do about it, and (3) that we have the power to act preventively. By failing to act until children and adolescents are damaged, we are dehumanizing children from a position of adult superiority that could be—but is not—used to protect them.

Another kind of exploitation that ignores children's developmental needs and opportunities is giving a higher priority to the paid work of mothers than to the unpaid work of nurturing their babies. State welfare-to-work policies can require a mother to return to work after her baby is 6 weeks old even though childcare at that age costs more than parental care and the income generated by parental employment. This makes the maternal care and breastfeeding of newborn babies less expensive than childcare. This juvenile ageist policy underlines the belief that paid work is more important to society than unpaid parenting even when its costs taxpayers more.

In her book *What Money Can't Buy*, Susan Mayer (1997) points out that the first rule of policy-making should be do not promulgate a policy that will interfere with social bonding. Still, a higher priority is given in public policies to parents working and paid childcare than to attachment bonding. Paid work is more highly valued even when a policy incurs higher immediate- and long-term costs for taxpayers. Because such a policy costs more, it is not based on economics. Instead, it reflects a prejudice against mothers who are receiving welfare and want to meet the developmental needs of their babies, as if mothering is not essential for their babies. This prejudice extends to employed mothers and fathers who do not have paid parental leaves as well.

6.4   Children as Commodities

In another vein, artificial insemination and childbearing are colored by the assumption that children are commodities. Embryos and fetuses are referred to as the "products of conception." Many workers, including laboratory technicians, physicians, lawyers and surrogate mothers, labor in this industry that produces and markets these human commodities.

The production of a baby through in vitro fertilization can involve five separate persons: the female genitor, the male genitor, the female surrogate, the functional mother, and the functional father. Each person brings new rights and duties to an enterprise in which the interests of the potential children are seldom considered. Accordingly, the state of Victoria in Australia was the first common-law jurisdiction to regulate infertility technologies. The Supreme Court of France outlawed surrogate motherhood entirely, holding that it violates a woman's body and undermines adoption.

In the United States, surrogacy is largely unregulated. In her New York Times article "Building a Baby with Few Ground Rules," Stephanie Saul (2009) called attention to the emerging commercial market for surrogate babies. Vexing ethical questions are raised. As a result, the American Bar Association has developed a model act for state legislatures. One section of the proposal holds that when prospective surrogate mothers have no genetic link to the babies, court pre-approval, including a home study, would be required.

Meanwhile, being admitted to California's Cryobank as a sperm donor is like getting into Harvard. The bank accepts fewer than 1% of its 26,000 applicants every year. One donor Googled his donor number. After locating a baby generated from his sperm, he sold a photo of the child to Cryobank for $200 so they could show how his offspring would look. The mother of that baby had already located two other babies. An impromptu online community of mothers who had used his sperm formed. As his sperm sold out quickly, he received $10,000 for each contribution.

A recent documentary on the Style network featured a donor who knows of at least 70 offspring from his donations. The implications for the scores of biologically related children and donors who can easily find each other have not been considered. In an Institute for American Values study My Daddy's Name Is Donor: A New Study of Young Adults Conceived through Sperm Donation (Clark et al. 2010), 45% of the resulting children felt bothered by the circumstances of their conception and that money was exchanged in order to conceive them.

In her book *The Revolution in Parenthood: The Emerging Global Clash between Adult Rights and Children's Needs*, Elizabeth Marquardt (2006) points out that when society changes marriage, it also changes parenthood. The divorce revolution and the rise in single-parent childbearing weakens father-child ties and introduces a host of rotating players called parents. The assisted reproductive technologies first used by married heterosexual couples and later by singles and same-sex couples raise still more uncertainties. The true meaning of motherhood and fatherhood comes into question, and children are exposed to new stressors and losses the adults never foresaw. The interests and rights of children are ignored … even possibly deliberately dismissed.

6.5 Where Are We Going?

Juvenile ageism permits us to have laws and social policies in which the loving, competent mother-father model is being replaced with the idea that babies, children, and adolescents can do well with any caregivers … after all they can and must adapt to our adult world. This idea flies in the face of the developmental needs and rights of children described later in Chap. 8 but first brings us to juvenile ageism in American society.

References

Clark, K., Glenn, N., & Marquardt, E. (2010). *My Daddy's name is donor: A pathbreaking new study of young adults conceived through sperm donation.* New York: Institute for American Values. http://www.americanvalues.org/search/item.php?id=25. Accessed 6 July 2018.

Marquardt, E. (2006). *The revolution in parenthood: The emerging global clash between adult rights and children's needs*. New York: Institute for American Values.

Mayer, S. (1997). *What money can't buy: Family income and children's life chances*. Cambridge, MA: Harvard University.

Saul, S. (2009, December 12). Building a baby, with few ground rules. *The New York Times*. https://www.nytimes.com/2009/12/13/us/13surrogacy.html. Accessed 6 July 2018.

Chapter 7
Categories of Juvenile Ageism

My own personal view, as a magistrate, is that our society intervenes far too late in the process of antisocial behavior as this develops in children. It is much easier, and more viable, to make rules in the homes and at school and enforce these, than to try rehabilitation programs on adults whose lives have been ruined by society's unwillingness to get involved until it is too late for the life habit of crime to be reversed.

Magistrate Sybil Eysenck (Eysenck, Gudjonsson et al. 1991)

The categories of ingrained societal juvenile ageism are:

1. When children are ignored as citizens with developmental needs as important as the needs and desires of adults
2. When children are unnecessarily segregated from public places and public media
3. When adolescents are treated as adults
4. When childcare systems do not serve the interests of children
5. When child development research is biased against the developmental needs of children
6. When public programs place parental wishes above children's interests

7.1 Ageism That Ignores Children as Citizens

The fact that debates occur over whether or not children are full-fledged citizens is a reflection of juvenile ageism. Children do not vote, and families with children are a minority in our society. Therefore, it is difficult for our political system to address their fundamental needs and problems. Our political system inherently tends to discriminate against children because they are not effectively represented. Parents do not have an extra vote for each child. Our political system discriminates against our children when its superior power advances adult interests while ignoring our responsibility to protect and further the interests of our children…our posterity as the next generation.

© Springer Nature Switzerland AG 2019
J. C. Westman, *Dealing with Child Abuse and Neglect as Public Health Problems*, https://doi.org/10.1007/978-3-030-05897-5_7

Prejudice and discrimination are fostered by the dominance of self-centered individualism and consumerism in our society. Encouraging financial success without concern for the well-being of others breeds self-indulgence and exploitation. The short-term satisfaction of personal desires takes an increasing priority over long-term commitments to spouses and to parenthood. The young are seen as burdens or exploitable consumers rather than as the next generation.

A prime example of the impact of individualism on families comes from childless taxpayers. They argue that child tax deductions unfairly shift the tax burden to them. One taxpayer without children complained, "I have been working since I was fifteen to support myself and am sick of families receiving aid." Another taxpayer said, "Those with more children use more services and should be taxed more heavily, rather than given a tax break."

Whenever the interests of adults and children conflict, adult interests almost always prevail, as if children are not citizens of equal standing. Unlike other minority or oppressed groups, children cannot claim their rights. In its 1977 publication, *All Our Children: The American Family under Pressure*, the Carnegie Council on Children presciently declared:

> …until policy makers and planners shift their focus to the broad ecological pressures on children and their parents, our public policies will be unable to do much more than help individuals repair the damage that environment is constantly re-inflicting on them.

Then as today virtually the last question we ask of any public policy is how it will affect our children. It should be the first question. *Eugene Steuerle, an economist with the Urban Institute, points out that our* nation's budget reflects priorities in which children, investment, and, more generally, our posterity rank low. *The interests of children are inevitably neglected* in budgetary crossfires (Carasso et al. 2007).

The Brookings Institution and Urban Institute's *Report on Federal Expenditures on Children Through 2010* projected that the children's share of the federal budget would drop from 11% to 8% in 2020 as mandated spending rises, especially for Social Security and Medicare (Isaacs et al. 2011).

These trends will aggravate the current plight of our children and youth that was predicted in the 1989 Report of the US Select Committee on Children, Youth, and Families. Two years later, the National Commission on Children pointed out "that the most prosperous nation in the world seems to be failing its children." The generally low priority set by federal, state, and county funding for vulnerable children, especially those who have been damaged by neglect and abuse, is a glaring example of societal juvenile ageism.

The associate director of the Milwaukee Department of Human Services pointed out to me that it is easier to get money for a penguin exhibit at the zoo than for child protection. For each $10.00 of Milwaukee County property taxes, the park system receives $2.01, the museum $0.36, the zoo $0.15, the performing arts center $0.12, the symphony $0.07, and child protection services $0.04. There are "friends" of museums and "friends" of zoos at budget appropriation hearings, but there are no "friends" of abused and neglected children.

Another example of ignoring the direct impact adult affairs have on children occurs when their interests are not considered sufficiently during divorce proceedings. Many children become victims of inadequate and unpaid child support. The moral and legal obligation of parents to financially support their children is ignored when those obligations are treated the same as unpaid credit card debts. The lack of enforcement amounts to societal support of child neglect. This has been recognized by the recent federal requirement that states vigorously enforce child support obligations.

7.2 Ageism That Segregates Children

The most pervasive form of societal juvenile ageism is the exclusion of children from public aspects of our society. Obviously, children and adults live in different worlds. Children's worlds are defined by their parents and the limited range of their environments. Children, therefore, can be denied access to a private adult world. Parents can restrict access to their bedrooms. Society also can designate certain places as adult-only. However, it does not follow that children should be denied access to public places or media that should be accessible to all citizens regardless of race, creed, gender, or age.

In order to protect children from unsafe public places and from the undesirable influences of movies, television programs, and magazines, certain public aspects of society are off limits to children. The emphasis is on excluding children from harmful influences rather than on creating a society in which children can freely participate. When we define our tolerance of public behavior, we act as though children are not members of the public. We set limits of tolerance according to the lowest adult standards rather than standards appropriate for children. We act as if children do not exist.

This exclusion means that children are denied free access to public places, public information, and public entertainment so that adults can have free access to activities that are harmful to children. The Constitutional right to free expression by adults often is pitted successfully against the need to protect children from pornography and violent images, as if children did not have rights. Instead of designating private places and media for adults, we segregate one-quarter of the population from public places and media. In effect, we create an unnecessarily segregated world for children.

Rather than creating a society with a suitable public atmosphere for our young citizens, parents are expected to protect and segregate their children from unsuitable public influences. In 2009, the US Supreme Court refused to hear an appeal of the 2000 Third Circuit Court of Appeals Decision in ACLU v. Reno II. The case blocked enforcement of the Child Online Protection Act, which established criminal penalties for online commercial distribution of material harmful to minors. The Appeals Court held that the Act was unconstitutional because it made every web communication provider abide by the most restrictive community's standards. Our societal, community, and media standards would be quite different if all adults, including the justices of the US Supreme Court, seriously considered how they are modeling values and behavior for our young citizens. Children and youth are watching all of us.

The rational that children should be segregated from unsafe places and undesirable public media rather than having society accommodate them was used to segregate women from the freewheeling "man's world." Fortunately, segregation and harassment of women in the armed forces and the workplace are no longer publicly tolerated. Both are expected to respectfully accommodate women. The same could be accomplished for children.

The segregation of children and youth can be compared to the same form of discrimination against adults. How would you respond to restricting the access of Black adults, women, homosexuals, or the physically handicapped to publicly sanctioned information, entertainment, and events that were offensive or harmful to them? Few people would tolerate this, yet we tolerate, condone, and promote events and materials that are offensive and harmful to one-quarter of our population... children and youth.

The only reasonable conclusion is that children are being treated as inferior beings rather than as citizens with age-appropriate rights comparable to those of adults. The most obvious consequence is the struggle of parents against violent and sexually stimulating societal influences. They are expected to protect their children from those public influences. They also are expected to gird their children against the dangers of public places and neighborhoods.

The most important example of self-destructive, societal juvenile ageism is indifference to the deteriorating quality of life of disadvantaged children and adolescents followed by punishing them for their behavior generated by incompetent parents and our society's failure to provide safe neighborhoods and schools. Our society has abandoned its role in protecting its young citizens. Except in rural and suburban areas, most children have lost the freedom of movement and association provided by safe neighborhoods. Neighborhoods have been disrupted by crime and social engineering. The main response of our policies has been to transfer childcare from home and neighborhood settings to institutions designed for custodial, safety, and educational purposes.

One such policy is found in the movement for daycare. The claim is that daycare centers are superior to parent care because they can take advantage of the latest innovations in education and child psychology. However professional segregation deprives them of the experiences that appear when people take responsibility for each other simply because they live in the same communities. In her book *Death and Life of Great American Cities,* Jane Jacobs (1961) suggested:

> The myth that playgrounds and grass and hired guards or supervisors are innately wholesome for children and that the city streets filled with ordinary people are innately evil for children, boils down to a deep contempt for ordinary people (and for children).

Many aspects of our society and its environments are not fit for children. Usually this obvious fact is minimized because the interests of children are not important enough to influence our social conduct. Instead, we uphold the myth that we will do anything for our children. In truth, we are more like a society that will do anything to our children.

If our society respected its immature members, we would ensure the safety of children in their neighborhoods. We would support parents' efforts to rear their children rather than accepting and even promoting public influences that are harmful to children.

7.3   Ageism That Treats Children as Adults

Perhaps surprisingly, juvenile ageism is expressed when children are treated as adults. In 1981 in *The Hurried Child*, psychologist David Elkind (2001) called attention to our society's trend toward regarding childhood and adolescence as stages of life to be outgrown as rapidly as possible (Elkind 2001). The philosopher Michael McFall (2009) in his book *Licensing Parents* details the ways in which adolescents are being treated as adults to their detriment today.

7.3.1   Prematurely Awarding Adult Responsibilities

By placing adult responsibilities on them prematurely, children are expected to be independent at the expense of their developmental needs. This occurs when children must adjust to adults' personal problems, work schedules, and lifestyles. It occurs when children are expected to raise younger siblings. It also occurs when children are expected to perform like adults in school and in athletics at ever earlier ages.

In her book *Ready or Not,* Kay Hymowitz (2000) exposes the fallacious belief that socializing children is a wrongful use of power and that children should develop on their own. This fallacy has been reinforced by writers such as Judith Harris (1998) who implied that parents are less important than peers in her book *The Nurture Assumption*, a view that was brilliantly debunked in just a few paragraphs by Denis Donovan and Deborah McIntyre (1999) in their book *What Did I Just Say!?!* (for an important real-world application of Donovan's critique of Harris' group socialization theory of development, see Donovan 2000). Peers do outweigh parents on fashions and attitudes, but parents are the dominant influences on character development. The presumption that children will socialize themselves is false. It treats them like adults before they have adult capacities.

A dramatic example of treating an adolescent as an adult occurred in the Netherlands in 2009. A Dutch court blocked would-be-record-breaking 13-year-old Laura Dekker from a 2-year solo sailing trip around the world. Intervening at the request of child protective services, the court put her under temporary supervision for 2 months to determine if she could withstand the physical and emotional risks. The fact that a court would even consider the adventure means it was open to treating a teenager as an adult.

7.3.2 Applying Punitive Adult Policies

Misbehaving children typically are met with punitive measures in line with a "get tough on crime" public approach to adult offenders. Recent decades have seen a trend toward reacting to the "children and youth crisis" with immediate zero-tolerance interventions. This view considers youth as the cause of crises rather than their families, neighborhoods, schools, and society. The emphasis is on "get tough" policies rather than society's failure to provide safe homes and neighborhoods or to model personal responsibility.

In his book *Framing Youth: 10 Myths about the Next Generation*, Mike Males (1999) noted that the deteriorating behavior of American grownups in both personal and social realms has led to youth becoming the target of displaced anxiety and fury. He said, "when America's elders screw up big time, expect them to trash the younger generation with a vengeance."

Strategies commonly used by schools are suspension, expulsion, and zero-tolerance policies that are reactive to behavior rather than dealing with the underlying causes. They presume that if youth know about harsh punishments, they will be less inclined to misbehave. Children and adolescents now are arrested and criminalized for behavior that once was dealt with by principals or guidance counselors. They are being shifted from the educational to the juvenile justice system. There they may well be passed on to the adult correctional system where they become hardened criminals. Rebellious children are behaving irrationally in our view as we overlook the fact that they live in struggling, confusing families. Many are attracted to antisocial gangs in spite of, and some because of, our punitive policies. The bigger the crime, the higher the status in gangs.

7.3.3 Requiring Children to Testify in Adult Courtrooms

Until the 1980s, sexually abused children were traumatized by having to testify in court. Eventually their immaturity and vulnerability were recognized, and appropriate interviewing technologies were developed. Despite this awareness, children still can be required to testify in court rooms.

A lawyer from the Los Angeles Chapter of the organization Victims of Child Abuse Legislation said, "They're always trying to throw away the Bill of Rights to protect children." This statement opposed legislation that would recognize that children are not adults and need special consideration in legal matters. The implication was that the Bill of Rights applies to adults but not to children.

7.3.4 Treating Children and Adolescents as Independent Persons

Systems that serve children often treat them as freestanding persons. When they are not treated as dependent parts of a parent-child unit, interventions actually can harm them. Proof of this abounds when adolescents are treated as adults in juvenile and criminal courts.

The limitations of the juvenile justice system illustrate how systems designed to protect and help young persons have the opposite effect when they ignore their families. In the In re Gault ruling in 1967, the US Supreme Court found it necessary to protect children from inappropriate placements away from home by courts. Even that decision can aggravate situations by focusing attention on procedural due process for minors as if they are not part of a child-parent unit. When this happens, children and their parents are further removed from appropriate help.

7.3.5 Adolescent Childbearing

As long ago as 1987, the Committee on Child Development Research and Public Policy of the National Research Council concluded that the lack of a coherent policy toward adolescent pregnancy and childbearing contributed to the magnitude and seriousness of the problem (Policy Institute 1990). The Committee found that adolescent parenthood is a handicap because it interferes with development and opportunities in life. The Committee emphasized postponing sexual intercourse until both males and females are capable of wise and responsible decisions.

Although the rate of adolescent childbirth has been decreasing, the numbers remain unacceptably high. At the present time, 2.6 million children have been born to mothers under the age of 18, roughly 145,000 each year. Over 234,000 babies were born to 18- and 19-year-olds in 2011. A significant proportion of the next generation that will need to cope with an ever more demanding and competitive society is being raised by adolescents with their parents or likely alone if they are over 18.

Solutions have been stymied because of the characteristics of adolescence and because too many adolescents want to have babies. Finding solutions is a formidable task in our society that prizes personal privacy and individual freedom and that broadly interprets reproductive freedom.

Rather than modeling self-restraint, the media exposes American adolescents to the most self-defeating of all possible messages. Sexual intercourse often is depicted as an activity with little mention of its risks or responsibilities. Nonmarital sex is portrayed as exciting. Little informs adolescents about the consequences of sexual activity or the realities of childrearing.

Moreover, children see premarital sex, cohabitation, and multiple sexual relationships among the adults they know, including their own parents. Few if any other societies exhibit a more confusing combination of permissiveness and prudishness. The mixed messages result in an adolescent childbirth rate from two to seven times that of comparable nations.

As it now stands, biological and social pressures encourage rather than discourage adolescent pregnancies. Since the brain does not fully mature until the third decade of life, the ability to procreate is present long before the cognitive, emotional, and social maturity required for parenthood. The average onset of menses at 12, earlier initiation of sexual intercourse, and intense social and peer pressures abetted by the commercial exploitation of sexuality are powerful forces that promote teen pregnancy.

Many adolescents are wishful thinkers. Their sense of invulnerability and their attraction to risk mean they believe "it can't happen to me." This underlies the "I don't care about that now" attitude despite knowing that cigarettes, drugs, noise, and steroids produce disease, addiction, deafness, and a shorter life span. Monitoring the Future surveys conducted by the Survey Research Center at the University of Michigan from 2001 to 2004 illuminate this attitude (ISR n.d.). For 56% of high school seniors, having a child outside of marriage was considered a worthwhile lifestyle or was thought not to affect anyone else.

Even more importantly, babies and young children need to be protected from these characteristics. Immaturity is inherent in adolescence and cannot be eliminated by persuasion or education. Adolescents need competent parents and a society that supports self-restraint. Yet those who are most likely to become pregnant are seldom exposed to values and experiences that reveal the disadvantages of adolescent childbirth. Even with that knowledge, a substantial number of adolescents ignore it.

Usually we direct solutions at adolescents as if they were independent persons. We advocate sex education, the availability of contraceptives, parenting training, supportive education, welfare payments, and expanded health care. None of those measures keep personal, educational, occupational, and developmental opportunities from disappearing. We cannot expect family-life education, school-based health clinics, and "increased life options" programs to change sexual behaviors and attitudes acquired through developmentally inappropriate sexual socialization or sexual abuse.

Our society's failure to deal with adolescent childbirth actually is a type of sexism against females, ageism against adolescents, and racism against minorities. The combined force of these prejudices and discrimination is seen most poignantly with the Black adolescent girl whose disadvantaged status is perpetuated when she is (1) impregnated to prove a "player's" masculinity (sexism), (2) deprived of the opportunity to complete her adolescent development (juvenile ageism), and (3) publicly viewed as following her cultural heritage and destiny (racism).

If we truly wish to prevent adolescent pregnancies and childbirth, we need to recognize that developmental characteristics and parental influences, or the lack thereof, are more important than ignorance and socioeconomic disadvantage. Anti-poverty measures alone will not address key parent-child relationship problems. Ronald Mincy and Susan Weiner (1990) of the Urban Institute found that poverty is less important than the parents in an adolescent girl's chances of becoming pregnant.

The focus also needs to extend to boys and young men. As long as boys fail to postpone fatherhood until they have steady employment and as long as men do not support their children, mothers and children will remain trapped in poor neighborhoods where social problems incubate and human services are ineffective.

Unfortunately, efforts to reduce adolescent pregnancy encounter powerful resistances. One is the belief that public attitudes toward irresponsible sexual behavior cannot be changed. Therefore, when pregnancy occurs, the focus is on pregnancy termination or on supporting the adolescent during pregnancy and while raising the child. Heated arguments revolve around notifying an adolescent's parents about the pregnancy as well as termination. Seldom are questions raised about the adolescents' ability to make life-altering decisions or their ability to rear children. Another resistance arises from the emphasis on a fetus's right to life that does not include the right of fetuses to competent parents after birth.

Our society cannot afford to shortchange the nurturing and protection of its immature members by allowing them to assume adult responsibilities. If we define parenthood as an adult responsibility, we can restore adolescence as a developmental stage of life for pregnant adolescents.

7.4 Juvenile Ageism in Childcare Systems

When managing the lives of children is turned over to impersonal institutions, adverse consequences can result. Institutions have considerations that might not reflect the interests of the children they serve.

Social service, correctional, legal and mental health institutions occupy established slots in our economy. They are as dependent on their clients as their clients are upon them. This does not mean that professionals intend to promote the continuation of the problems they are supposed to solve. But institutional factors like the lack of interagency collaboration, budget cuts, and protecting budgetary turfs can stall them at the level of servicing rather than solving economic, social, and family problems.

Policies and practices reflect inadvertent juvenile ageism when children are treated impersonally and categorically. For example, two blanket social services policies override the interests of individual children. The first is the child protection policy that removes children from abusive parents. When the child removal policy dominates, children can be taken from their homes and placed in foster care indefinitely. The conditions that led to their removal may never be addressed effectively. The second is the family preservation policy meant to maintain existing family structures. Because of the shortage of effective services and the failure to follow statutory requirements, this policy can keep children in, and return children to, families that further damage them. Instead of adhering to blanket policies, the needs of each child and family should determine how best to help that child.

Similarly, public schools have long been used to achieve sociopolitical aims such as crime prevention, poverty amelioration, and racial integration. Each goal might be laudable, but each one can deflect attention from the developmental needs of the young and the vital role of parent-child relationships in those social problems.

In addition, public school teachers generally are underpaid, leading to strikes in schools aimed at increasing their salaries to a more appropriate level. Childcare works also are underpaid.

Moreover, services meant to benefit children can serve the interests of those who provide them instead. For example, the primary role of childcare systems is to serve the adults who delegate childcare to others and those who provide the childcare rather than the interests of the children themselves.

Another example can be found in federal regulations that mandate costly treatment for every newborn not born dead. This is done without regard for the newborn's quality of life or the baby's family. No financial provisions are provided once these severely handicapped, technologically dependent babies leave neonatal intensive care. Since their families are financially and emotionally stressed and the children do not have a fully conscious life, the quality of their families' lives, including that of their siblings, is grossly impaired.

7.5   Juvenile Ageism in Child Development Research

As David Hamburg (1992, 2011), Executive Director of the Carnegie Foundation, pointed out in The Family Crucible and Healthy Child Development, newborns in the United States are treated like experimental subjects. We expose them to an unlimited variety of parents until they are damaged by neglect and abuse. Then we study them to see what kind of parenting they had.

More specifically, the way questions are framed in child development research can reflect juvenile ageism. This prejudice underlies resiliency research that assesses how much neglect and abuse or how much placement in nonfamilial environments young children can tolerate without being permanently damaged. Compare this once again to research on how much neglect and abuse or how much segregation Jews, Blacks or elders could tolerate without being seriously damaged to bring the prejudice into clear view.

Research on child neglect and abuse usually asks whether actions and practices harm children rather than whether they are in the developmental interests of children. Even though adult women are readily designated as victims of domestic abuse on the basis of their complaints, children often are not considered victims of abuse unless they are obviously damaged by it. Instead of assuming that they need competent parents, the assumption is that they are not harmed by their parents unless serious damage can be proved. The research, therefore, focuses on the resilience of neglected and abused children rather than on the children's developmental interests in the quality of their parenting.

In a similar vein, research on the effects of parental prenatal substance abuse assesses the extent of damage to children later in life. The ongoing Maternal

Lifestyle Study conducted at four NICHD Neonatal Research Network sites found in 2008 that the damage is less than previously thought (NICHD 2008). Along with declining rates of adolescent pregnancy and alcohol and substance abuse, these findings are used to reduce the importance of these problems as if there is an acceptable level of damage to children.

Other studies are similarly flawed. Research on the effects of childcare on children usually takes for granted the unavailability of parents employed away from home and does not ask how much nonparental care is in the developmental interests of the children or the parents. Criminology research focuses on children as offenders—delinquents—rather than as victims of adversity.

When the emphasis of research is on assessing how much children are harmed by incompetent parents, maternal prenatal drug use, and separation from their parents, a child's need for competent parents is not taken into account.

7.6   When Public Programs Place Parental Wishes Above Children's Interests

The following article in the Tampa Bay Times about the work of a Florida task force devoted to "helping babies in drug withdrawal" through Neonatal Abstinence exemplifies the way in which a narrow focus on a specific problem obscures the big picture and results in continuing newborn babies in circumstances that are contrary to their interests:

> Sarah Ryan had previously lost custody of her three sons in the context of her long-standing battle with drug addiction. When she became pregnant again she was "petrified to actually tell a physician that I was addicted, because I didn't want to lose my child." She finally did tell her doctor and was put on methadone during the last trimester of pregnancy. When born her baby Quinn seemed healthy, but on his third day he began to show signs of methadone withdrawal. He was placed on methadone and then weaned over 3 ½ weeks in intensive care. Ryan now is caring for her healthy baby and receiving treatment through the Tampa Drug Abuse Comprehensive Coordinating Office. (Stein 2013)

In this example, the narrow focus on the wishes of a mother and on the condition of a newborn baby completely ignored the fact that this mother had been found to be an unfit parent for three previous children. Instead of seeking a pre-emptive termination of parental rights based on her history and the fact of neonatal child abuse through the use of drugs, the point was that more research is called for to identify the best way to treat newborns in withdrawal. The goal of the task force is "not to arrest mothers and take their babies away from mothers. It's to prevent this (babies in drug withdrawal) from happening." It is not a stretch to see this attitude as deferring to the wishes of mothers and viewing their newborn babies as their property rather than as persons with rights and interests of their own…as an expression of juvenile ageism.

7.7   Where Are We?

In all of these systems that presumably are intended to help our young citizens, the failure of professionals and their funders to make corrections in policies and practices in the face of demonstrated harm to our youngest children makes inadvertent juvenile ageism more sinister. A prominent example is found in the "war against child abuse." In some respects, it has become a war against children who become its casualties when they are treated solely as individuals rather than as part of a child/parent unit in a family that is crying out for help. This brings us to the ways in which juvenile ageism harms our young citizens.

References

Carasso, A., Reynolds, G., & Steuerle, C. E. (2007). *How much does the federal government spend to promote economic mobility and for whom?* (Economic Mobility Project). Philadelphia: Pew Charitable Trusts. https://www.urban.org/sites/default/files/publication/31456/411610-how-much-does-the-federal-government-spend-to-promote-economic-mobility-and-for-whom-.pdf. Accessed 6 July 2018.

Donovan, D. M. (2000). Rethinking adoption. *Adoption/Medical News, 6*(9–10), 1–11. Reprinted in Thomas C. Atwood (ed.), *Adoption Factbook IV*. Alexandria, VA: National Council for Adoption.

Donovan, D. M., & McIntyre, D. (1999). *What did I just say!?! How new insights into childhood thinking can help you communicate with your child from infancy through adolescence* (pp. 164–166). New York: Henry Holt & Company.

Elkind, D. (2001). *The hurried child: Growing up too fast too soon.* New York: Perseus.

Eysenck, H. J., & Gudjonsson, G. H. (1991). *The causes and cures of criminality* (pp. 7–8). New York: Plenum Press.

Hamburg, D. A. (1992). *Today's children: Creating a future for a generation in crisis.* New York: Times Books, Random House.

Hamburg, D. A. (2011). *The family crucible.* New York: The Carnegie Corporation. https://files.eric.ed.gov/fulltext/ED353037.pdf. Accessed 6 July 2018.

Harris, J. R. (1998). *The nurture assumption: Why children turn out the way they do.* New York: The Free Press.

Hymowitz, K. (2000). *Ready or not: Why treating children as small adults endangers their future.* New York: Encounter Books.

Isaacs, J., et al. (2011). *Kid's share: Report on federal expenditures on children through 2010.* Washington, DC: Brookings, the Urban Institute. https://www.brookings.edu/wp-content/uploads/2016/06/0721_kids_share_isaacs.pdf. Accessed 6 July 2018.

ISR [Institute for Social Research]. (n.d.). University of Michigan. https://www.icpsr.umich.edu/icpsrweb/ICPSR/series/35. Accessed 6 July 2018.

Jacobs, J. (1961). *Death and life of great American cities.* New York: Random House.

Males, M. (1999). *Framing youth: 10 myths about the next generation.* Monroe: Common Courage Press.

McFall, M. (2009). *Licensing parents: Family, state, and child maltreatment.* New York: Lexington Books.

Mincy, R. B., & Wiener, S. J. (1990). *A mentor, peer group, incentive model for helping underclass youth* (Research Paper). Washington, DC: Urban Institute. https://files.eric.ed.gov/fulltext/ED337524.pdf. Accessed 6 July 2018.

NICHD [National Institute of Child Health and Human Development]. (2008, September). Pregnancy and Perinatology Branch (PPB). Report to the NACHHD Council. https://www1. nichd.nih.gov/publications/pubs/Documents/ppb_council_2008_historical.pdf. Accessed 6 July 2018.

Policy Institute for Family Impact Seminars, Purdue University. (1990). Evolving state policies on teen pregnancy and parenthood: What more can the feds do to help? https://www.purdue.edu/ hhs/hdfs/fii/wp-content/uploads/2015/06/pf_fis15report.pdf. Accessed 6 July 2018.

Stein, L. (2013, February 9). State wants to help newborns withdrawing from moms' pain pill addiction. *Tampa Bay Times*. http://www.tampabay.com/news/health/state-wants-to-help-new-borns-withdrawing-from-moms-pain-pill-addiction/1274593. Accessed 5 June 2018.

Chapter 8
The Impact of Juvenile Ageism on Individuals

We are always too busy for our children. We never give them the time or interest they deserve. We lavish gifts upon them, but the most precious gift – our personal association, which means so much to them – we give grudgingly and throw it away on those who care for it so little.

Mark Twain

Ageism against an individual child disregards that child as a person without moral and civil rights. The most extreme form is seen in the belief that parents own their children as property. This was reflected in a letter circulated by the National Parents' Survey on Public Education:

Dear Friend:
Who owns your children?
Who decides what values, attitudes, and beliefs they should hold?
Is it you–the parent?
Or is it government through the public education system? (Bowman 2012)

8.1 Children as Property

The belief that children are the property of their parents draws upon the deeply ingrained assumption that genetic parents have natural affection for their offspring and that parenthood is a reproductive right. It is supported by the legal presumption that others can interfere with parental authority only when parents seriously damage children through neglect or abuse.

There is another side of this coin. The ambivalent emotions inherent in all parent-child relationships are depicted in the Oedipus complex. In Sophocles' tragedy Oedipus Rex, his mother Jocasta arranges to have 3-day-old Oedipus killed because she fears he will ultimately kill her husband. As an adult, Oedipus discovers this from a servant:

© Springer Nature Switzerland AG 2019
J. C. Westman, *Dealing with Child Abuse and Neglect as Public Health Problems*, https://doi.org/10.1007/978-3-030-05897-5_8

OEDIPUS: You mean she gave the child to you?
SERVANT: Yes, my lord.
OEDIPUS: Why did she do that?
SERVANT: So I would kill it.
OEDIPUS: That wretched woman (his wife) was the mother?
SERVANT: Yes. She was afraid of dreadful prophecies.
OEDIPUS: What sort of prophecies?
SERVANT: The story went that he would kill his father.

After this revelation, Jocasta commits suicide, and Oedipus, who has mistakenly married his mother and killed his father, blinds himself and becomes homeless. Both mother and son suffer from their beliefs and actions. Sophocles dramatically calls attention to the conflicting feelings, motives, and actions naturally involved to a less intense degree in parent-child relationships. This ambivalence is fertile soil for prejudice and discrimination when children are regarded as their parents' property.

At the deepest psychological levels, we cannot overlook the tradition of parents having total control over their children's lives … even the ability to abandon and kill them, as still is done in some parts of the world. The Biblical example of Abraham and Isaac illustrates the power of a parent over a child. Although the practice of child sacrifice was abandoned long ago, it continues to exert a powerful unconscious influence. The following examples demonstrate how this absolute control persists.

8.2   Killing a Child Is Not Murder

Homicide is the leading cause of death by injury for babies in the United States. Michael Petit (2011), President of Every Child Matters, pointed out in 2011 that over the previous 10 years, more than 20,000 American children were believed to have been killed in their own homes by family members. That was nearly four times the number of US soldiers killed in Iraq and Afghanistan during that time. The child maltreatment death rate in the United States triples Canada's and 11 times that of Italy. This number is low because between 60% and 85% of child fatalities due to maltreatment are not recorded as such on death certificates.

In New York City, a mother's drug abuse caused the premature birth and death of her child; the death was ruled as "natural causes" (Buder 1988). In Indiana, murder charges against Melody Baldwin were dropped when she pleaded guilty to child abuse after administering a fatal dose of a drug to her 4-year-old son (AP 1998). In Wisconsin, a judge remarked that the death by beating of a 20-month-old boy by his 26-year-old prostitute mother "may well have been a benevolent grace for the child" because of the sordid life that boy would otherwise have had to bear.

A more subtle but revealing sign of juvenile ageism is found in a New York City Child Fatality Report. Generally, the deaths of premature newborns caused by their mothers' drug abuse were noted as "deaths from natural causes" (Jenny and Isaac 2006).

Our society has a deep-seated respect for the mother-child relationship along with an understandable aversion to blaming parents. This is best illustrated by the public reaction that any mother who kills her children must be mentally ill (Register Staff 1993).

> A 29-year-old mother, Kimberly Martin, was charged with first degree murder in the deaths of 8-year-old Dusty and 4-year-old Brandy, whose bodies were found in her car when she was stopped for speeding in Council Bluffs, Iowa. Each child was shot in the head. The insanity of a mother who shot and killed her two young children appeared so clear-cut that neither the prosecution nor the judge required evidence that Martin was mentally ill at the time of the shootings. The judge found Kimberly Martin innocent by reason of insanity and released her from custody.

The fact that the victims were her own children allowed Martin's murders to be explained in a way that would be unacceptable if she had murdered two unrelated children. With the murder of adults, determining innocence by reason of insanity involves questions about premeditation, awareness of right and wrong, and the ability to adhere to the right. These questions used to determine insanity were not raised in Martin's case. The verdict also presumes that murdering her own children does not suggest that she might be dangerous to others as well.

What if Dusty and Brandy Martin had been killed by their father or a different relative? We cannot escape the possibility that the tradition of a child as a mother's property lies in the background of this and similar cases. The reluctance to believe that a mother could intentionally harm her child further confuses the issue. Latent guilt in those of us who are parents also could encourage us to deny the guilt of other parents.

The following note left by a mother who killed her daughter in St. Petersburg, Florida, before killing herself reveals the self-centered side of motherly love:

> I couldn't even take care of my daughter. I had to take her with me. I had no choice. I would not want her to go through her life without me in it.

8.3 Killing an Abusive Parent Is Murder

Killing your own parent cannot be excused under any circumstances. Still, a parent's superior power can goad a helpless, damaged child into the understandable response of attacking the abuser. Studies of adolescents who killed their parents reveal that many acted in self-defense. All of them released pent-up rage instilled by years of being battered. Slaves responded in similar ways to abusive masters.

One teenager who killed his abusive mother made the following comment:

> The biggest thing is just being aware. Care, 'cause if you don't, it's not just the little kid you are hurting, you're hurting tomorrow…. Because kids are defenseless, they don't have the vocabulary, the mental capacity, the mentality, the strong points to stand up. If someone won't stand up for them, nobody will. If no one does, then, what's tomorrow? (Heide 2013)

The view that parents who are killed by their children are victims while the victim status of their children is ignored betrays a prejudice against children. Of course, many adult murderers were neglected and abused as children. It is not that their crimes do not warrant prosecution. It is that as childhood victims of neglect and abuse our society did not value them enough to ensure adequate care for them. Thus, parents can be seen as victims of the children they have victimized. A society that accepts this formulation clearly discriminates against its young.

8.4   Exploitation of a Child

Children are particularly vulnerable to prejudice and discrimination in their own homes. They compete with their parents for time, money, attention, and affection. They require the compromise and sacrifice of adult wishes and needs. In response, many parents neglect their children or take out their frustrations on them. When children adapt to neglect or abuse, they are considered resilient.

> Katie Beers was called "the cockroach kid" in her neighborhood. At the age of 6, she was on the streets from dawn to darkness cutting her first-grade classes regularly. She survived as a Dickens street waif in a modern strip mall. At the age of 10, she came to the attention of authorities when she was found in a secret room underneath a Bay Shore home where she had been kept a prisoner by a family friend John Esposito. After closely reviewing their files, county social service officials believe they had handled the case properly before this discovery.

> Suffolk county Court Judge Joel Lefkowitz sentenced Esposito to a 15 years to life prison sentence for kidnapping. He also sentenced Sal Inghilleri, the husband of Katie's godmother, to a 14-year prison for sexually abusing Katie, saying Inghilleri had "robbed her of her youth." (UPI 1994)

The media coverage—40 articles in Newsday—portrayed Katie as a heroic figure, even a celebrity. She showed the qualities admired in adults...perseverance, adaptability, and an uncomplaining attitude that enabled her to surmount adversity. Her premature adulthood was seen as a virtue rather than as a defense against maltreatment. This view shifted attention away from the adults who mistreated her. The impact of interrupting her education, missing unencumbered play with peers, and future effects on her personality and social development was completely ignored.

Most significantly, depriving a child of the opportunity to live childhood as a developmental stage was not seen as the same as depriving adults of opportunities to fulfill their potential. Katie Beers was a victim of prejudice and discrimination by caretakers and a society that treats children as less important than adults. She was enslaved by parent figures, neglected by educational and social services and unprotected by society. In the end, she became a heroine, not a victim. This defensive distortion occurs regularly when survivors of child maltreatment are portrayed as heroic figures while attention is deflected away from their cruel treatment. Adults under the same circumstances would be considered victims of oppression and possibly torture who display the Stockholm syndrome.

In the movie Precious, an obese, poor, illiterate, young black woman who was sexually and emotionally abused becomes a heroine. A public relations specialist in Manhattan found it a "deeply moving way to show the beauty and innocence of a poor, fat, dark-skinned woman. At the end of the film, Precious looked angelic to me" (Lee 2009).

8.5   The Fetus Is a Mother's Property

There has been a long-standing legal tendency to regard an unborn child as part of the mother's body and, therefore, as her property. The limits of this belief were clarified in 1973 by the US Supreme Court ruling in Roe v. Wade that recognized the rights of a woman over the rights of the fetus during the first trimester, of the fetus over the mother in the second and third trimesters, and of a physician throughout pregnancy to make decisions regarding its termination.

The specification of maternal and fetal rights during pregnancy caused an abortion controversy that the US Supreme Court returned to state legislatures in Webster v. Reproductive Health Services in 1989. Because of this, the definition of ageism against a fetus remains to be clarified as our society defines its stand on abortion. In the medical community, the trend toward recognizing both the mother and an older fetus as separate patients has been prompted by surgery on a late-term fetus.

In another vein, the case of 17-year-old Jamine Bedwell illustrates how sympathy for an adolescent mother can obscure her parental incompetence even when it results in her baby's murder. The headline of one newspaper article was: "Mother Did Her Best for Infant: Officials Say the Teen Mother Tried to Keep Her Son Safe, But Could Not Stop Her Abusive Boyfriend."

Jasmine Bedwell's ex-boyfriend, 21-year-old Richard McTear, attacked her, drove off, and threw her baby Emanuel on to an interstate highway. Caught a few hours later, he was jailed facing 10 charges, including first-degree murder.

Tampa police records show Bedwell ran away from home at least 21 times. She was arrested 10 times, including a battery charge at the age of 11. Social workers intervened when she was 14. At 17, she gave birth to Emanuel. The father, Emanuel Murray, 22, was soon out of the picture, imprisoned on weapons charges.

McTear's record was filled with domestic violence arrests. McTear's beatings sent Bedwell to the hospital, according to a Department of Children and Families report. She went to court with a case worker to obtain an injunction against McTear whom process servers could not find. After 15 days, Bedwell did not pick up required paperwork. She did not attend a hearing several days later nor did McTear, who returned to her home to assault her and murder her baby.

Jeff Rainey, president and CEO of Hillsborough Kids Inc., a privately contracted child support service, said Bedwell did everything she could to protect Emanuel. (Jamison 2013)

The focus on the older man who repeatedly abused Bedwell and on her statement "I love my baby with all my heart, and he was the only thing I had left in life" ignores the fact that a baby was killed because of her ineptness as an adolescent. Emanuel's right to life was obscured. The support given to a troubled girl because she said she loved her baby despite the fact that her actions and inactions proved otherwise reflects two kinds of juvenile ageism. The first treats adolescents as adults. The second treats babies as objects whose only purpose is to fulfill their parents' needs.

8.6   The Baby Business

Parents across time have weighed the eventual economic contribution of their children in the rice field or the manor against the cost of raising them. They have used infanticide or abandonment to rid themselves of less-valued offspring. They also have sold them into slavery or indentured servitude.

Over the last 40 years, advances in reproductive medicine have created another market for babies. Affluent parents choose traits, clinics woo clients, and specialized providers earn millions of dollars a year. The typical costs of sperm are $300; eggs $4500; in vitro fertilization $67,000–$114,000 per live birth; surrogacy $59,000; adoption $2500 for a foster child, $15,000 for a domestic baby, and $25,000 for an international child; and preimplantation genetic diagnosis $3500. Physicians, who might charge over $10,000 for a procedure, need to answer a series of thorny ethical, safety, and social welfare questions.

Because few want to define baby-making as a business, and because the endeavor touches deeply on the most difficult moral dilemmas, many governments have either ignored this trade in children or simply prohibited it. An exception is that since 1991, the UK Human Fertilization and Embryology Authority has adopted rules for in vitro fertilization and embryo manipulation. In the United States, no binding rules deter a private clinic from offering a menu of sperm and egg traits or from implanting women with embryos.

In all of these instances, sperm, eggs, embryos, and fetuses are treated as commodities to be manipulated, bought, and sold without considering the consequences for the product…a human being. *Technology is forcing the legal system to define the fundamental meaning of parents, of a family, and of reproduction. It must consider current structures and develop new policy options for the marketplace, recipients, donors, and children, as well as the industry that serves them.*

In another vein in 2004, when Playtex débuted a breast pump called Embrace, no one pointed out that something you plug into a wall socket is a far cry from cuddling and a kiss. Pumps are a handy way to avoid the privately agonizing and publicly unpalatable question: Does the mother or her milk matter more to the baby? Many of breast-feeding's benefits come from the cuddling that accompanies it. The stark difference between employer-sponsored lactation programs and flesh-and-blood family life is difficult to overstate. Some lactation rooms even "ban babies lest mothers smuggle them in for a quick nip."

8.7 Irresponsible Artificial Fertilization

Some women choose to not have babies. Others exhaust every option to have a baby after they have been told they cannot give birth to one. Since the birth of the world's first "test-tube baby," Louise Brown in July 1978, the world has seen an estimated five million babies resulting from IVF and other assisted reproductive technologies, according to a presentation at the 2012 International Committee for Monitoring Assisted Reproductive Technologies (Bryner 2012).

Arthur Caplan (1986), bioethics chairman at the University of Pennsylvania, notes that not enough attention is paid to the well-being of the children in IVF-induced multiple births. Everyone has a stake in high-multiple births. They cause insurance premiums to rise when hospitals are not reimbursed properly. Those with disabilities typically require medical and social services. "To say all you need is cash and the will to have more kids should not be a sufficient standard to access fertility services," Caplan said. "It's insufficient for adoption. It isn't sufficient to be a foster parent. Why would it be sufficient to run down to the fertility clinic to get embryos transplanted or super-ovulated?"

Nadya Suleman, a 33-year-old single mother, already had six children, ages 2–7, when she gave birth to octuplets on January 26, 2009 (Debolt 2017). She had all 14 of her children through in vitro fertilization. She had been supporting herself in part on the more than $165,000 in disability payments she collected for a work injury and from $490 a month in food stamps. She had suffered bouts of paranoia and depression.

Suleman told NBC's Today she never stopped trying to get pregnant by fertility treatment to extend her family and make up for being an only child. "That was always a dream of mine, to have a large family, a huge family." She said that her childhood left her feeling a lack of self and identity. She was deluged with offers for book deals, TV shows, and other business proposals. Raina Kelley (2009), a Newsweek reporter, commented about what the outrage over Suleman says about our society:

> We created Octomom. Our democracy gives people the right to have as many children as they want. With our glorification of bizarre behavior, we dare the emotionally needy to shock and appall us. Then we slam them.

8.8 Fetal Damage Is Not the Responsibility of the Parent

In most states, whether a pregnant person's drug abuse constitutes child abuse is an open question. Still, some prosecutors, judges, and child-protection workers say they have an obligation to protect fetuses. The district attorney of California's Butte County vowed to seek jail terms for pregnant women who refuse to obtain treatment for drug abuse. Others say such action would create fetal rights that have no foundation in law.

In 1991, the Michigan Court of Appeals ruled that Kimberly Hardy, a 24-year-old factory worker, should not stand trial on child abuse charges for using crack hours before her son's birth. The child abuse statute did not apply to fetuses. On the other hand, in Westchester County, New York, a drug-abusing woman lost custody of her baby at birth after a judge ruled the child was likely to be neglected after birth.

In another case in Washington, DC, 29-year-old Brenda Vaughn pleaded guilty to forgery. Because tests showed that she had used cocaine, the Superior Court in the District of Columbia sent her to jail until her due date to protect the fetus from drug abuse. That case kindled heated debate about the use of child abuse and drug laws to prosecute illegal drug users and to place their newborns in foster care. Efforts to incarcerate pregnant drug addicts to prevent fetal damage have been criticized. The concern is that if a woman can be arrested for endangering a fetus with cocaine, she might be arrested for drinking alcohol or smoking. The failure to tie damage suffered by a fetus caused by the mother's behavior to a child's later disabilities clearly reflects juvenile ageism.

8.9   Abduction

The kidnapping of children by their parents is another example of children being regarded as possessions. Although the interests of children might be served by parental abduction at times, the most common cause is parents retaliating against each other.

Family violence might be involved in parental abduction. The abductor might be the violent one or the one fleeing violence. In other instances of abduction, parents ease their emotional pain despite the pain it causes the other parent or the confusion and stress experienced by the children. In any event, a child is being treated like an object to be possessed.

8.10   Removal from Adoptive Parents

Juvenile ageism exists when children's interests are disregarded by removing them from adoptive parents and returning them to incompetent genetic parents because of technical or legal errors in the adoption process. The child is treated as an object that can be readily moved from one place to another rather than as a human being with developmental needs and legal rights.

The case of In the Interests of J. L. W. is an example. In Wisconsin, a 5-month-old boy was abandoned by his mother (In Interest of LWJ 1981). When he was 18 months, parental rights were terminated, so he could be adopted by an aunt and uncle. Two years later, the state Supreme Court returned him to his genetic mother because of a technical error in the adoption rather than considering the child's circumstances and developmental interests in a new trial. The Court's order treated the child as an object and took him away from the only parents he knew.

In New Haven, Connecticut, a 1-year-old girl was returned to the 19-year-old mother who had abandoned her at birth. Five months after the termination of her parental rights, the mother asked to have her child returned. After legal action, the child was returned to her genetic mother without considering her attachment bonds with her adoptive parents, the only parents she knew.

In these cases, technical procedural issues forced the return of children to unfit parents. But when the legal issue actually hinges on genetic or psychological relationships between parents and children, the psychological relationship usually is considered paramount. In 1983, in Lehr v. Robertson, the US Supreme Court held that the emotional attachment, not the genetic relationship, defines the family (Lehr v. Robertson 1983).

8.11 Retrieval of Switched Baby

The belief that a child is the property of the genetic parents is further illustrated by the usual response to babies who are switched at birth. A Sarasota, Florida, couple tried to determine if their deceased 9-year-old daughter had been mistakenly switched at birth with another 9-year-old named Kimberly Mays in the hospital (Spargo 2015). They never considered the adverse effect such a pursuit might have on the living child. After one court granted them visitation rights on the basis of genetic testing, Kimberly fortunately was able to obtain a "divorce" from them in another court.

8.12 Corporal Punishment

Controversy over corporal punishment hinges on the fact that, although it is prohibited in many states' public schools, it has not been deemed by the US Supreme Court to be cruel and unusual punishment. Some people advocate corporal punishment because it is consistent with Biblical teachings. Others see any form of physical intervention as child abuse and the promotion of violence.

Those who advocate corporal punishment can use their beliefs to disguise child abuse. They might be reliving the violence they faced early in their lives. Those who oppose corporal punishment can use their beliefs to deprive children of useful lessons about the consequences of their behavior. Juvenile ageism is evidenced in both extremes. Realistic developmental interests are ignored when adults base their behavior on ideological beliefs rather than on the circumstances in which physical interventions are appropriate in the course of childrearing.

8.13   Animal Protection Has a Higher Priority

The way we protect animals dramatically contrasts with the way we protect children. Over 135 years of "child saving" has done little to reduce child neglect and abuse in the United States. The prevention of cruelty to animals, however, has been so successful that public protests against the use of animals in medical research are readily organized. Significantly, the formation of the New York Society for the Prevention of Cruelty to Children was preceded by a decade by the New York Society for the Prevention of Cruelty to Animals. The prevention of cruelty to animals is a familiar public theme. No so for the prevention of cruelty to children.

8.14   Responses of the Young to Juvenile Ageism

When young people internalize juvenile ageism, they often question their legitimacy, doubt their abilities, and perpetuate a culture of silence. They feel that they really do not count. They seek the approval of adults even if it means betraying other children by tattling on siblings or becoming a teacher's pet.

In a positive vein, discrimination against the young is increasingly recognized as bigotry around the world. The 2009 Portland National Youth Summit drafted a Mental Health Youth Bill of Rights (Strachan et al. 2009). An increasing number of social institutions are acknowledging children and youth as an oppressed minority group, especially when adolescents are generally characterized as immature, violent, and rebellious.

Psychotherapists, juvenile probation personnel, teachers, and other professionals have a special responsibility to avoid juvenile ageism by viewing young people as citizens with a right to participate in, and a responsibility to serve, their communities. Proponents of building on the strengths of young people through youth-adult partnerships and healthier communities offer a contrast to the view of the young as societal burdens that need to be controlled.

Curricula are available for educating adults about juvenile ageism. Organizations responding to the negative effects of juvenile ageism, including the United Nations in its Convention on the Rights of the Child (Articles 5 and 12), Human Rights Watch, the National Youth Rights Association, Youth on Board, and the Free Child Institute, envision a world in which young people are fully respected and treated as valued, active members of their families, communities, and society (UNICEF n.d.; HRW 2010; Youth On Board n.d.; FreeChild Institute n.d.).

Establishing and cultivating a productive, positive social climate requires adults and youth to take stock of their current beliefs. Adults need to exercise leadership roles in a spirit of service and respect especially when dealing with disrespectful youth. Young people need encouragement to assume responsibility for their own behavior and for learning.

8.15   Lack of Awareness of Juvenile Ageism

One reason why the elderly are more readily seen as victims of ageism than children is that most of us do not encounter egregious forms of juvenile ageism. We support public schools and child-oriented charities while disapproving of child neglect and abuse. Most children actually are valued and well-treated.

Our lack of awareness is understandable. First of all, juvenile ageism is eclipsed by our concern about racism and sexism. Second, we all are juvenile ageists to some degree. Third, we all have difficulty recognizing our prejudices even when they are pointed out to us. As much as we might like to believe otherwise, all of our judgments are biased by our experiences and our emotional states.

Juvenile ageism and other prejudices are easily obscured because they can be expressed in benevolent ways. Prejudice as an attitude and discrimination as a behavior are easier to recognize when they are expressed in malevolent ways. When children are oppressed, abused, and neglected, it is easier to accept the existence of juvenile ageism than when we believe we are helping and protecting them.

Making the case for juvenile ageism is a difficult task. In some ways, to speak of juvenile ageism now is like speaking about racism in the South in the 1850s. The economic interests and latent guilt of plantation owners kept them from recognizing slavery as a racist institution. Today, the latent guilt of adults and the commercial exploitation of the young keep us from recognizing juvenile ageism in our society and in our families.

8.16   What Does All of This Mean?

Because prejudice and discrimination are inherent in the human condition, active efforts are required to combat them. The concept of juvenile ageism helps us become aware that attitudes toward children can be prejudiced and that behavior toward children can be discriminatory. Juvenile ageism can be easily equated with elder ageism. Neglecting the interests of children because they are less important than and are inferior to adults is the same as neglecting the interests of persons whose race or gender is seen as relegating them to an inferior status.

Actually, juvenile ageism has the virulence of racism and the prevalence of sexism. It fosters the belief that parents can create and rear children without facing responsibilities to them or to society. It enables the exploitation, neglect, abuse, abduction, and even murder of children. It has contributed to the alienation of our youth from society's positive values. It is the greatest barrier to recognizing the interests of our young citizens in our political processes, in childcare systems and in households.

The consequences of juvenile ageism are a political system that fails to create safe environments for children, a commercial system that exploits the young, social services that are overwhelmed by child neglect and abuse cases, an impaired workforce, and a fragile economy. It has resulted in staggering costs from violence, habitual crime, and welfare dependency ... the ultimate products of child neglect and abuse.

Identifying and overcoming juvenile ageism requires a civil rights approach. If you feel hopeless about confronting or defeating juvenile ageism, you are confirming the ingrained power of this prejudice. Children should be recognized as citizens from birth. This means sensitizing the public to the existence of juvenile ageism and to the developmental requirements of childhood and adolescence.

Beyond that is the need for advocacy for newborns, children, and adolescents as well as their families. Of greatest importance is respect and support for the responsibilities of parenthood. Short-term sacrifices for long-term gain are politically unpopular in a society devoted to immediate gratification. Yet, the direct benefits to adults of a society in which children can thrive are reductions in crime, safe streets, integrity in commerce and politics, wholesome environments, and economic prosperity.

Overcoming juvenile ageism will benefit all adults and the next generation. Because it involves protecting our young and planning for the future, it is a theme around which improving our entire society can be organized. The immediate question is should we continue to expect children to cope with the stressors our society imposes on them? Juvenile ageism makes children responsible for coping with adult failings. Instead, we should minimize avoidable stressors for children and adolescents. This would emphasize our society's responsibility to protect and nurture our young citizens ... our next generation.

If juvenile ageism is not addressed, our nation is in peril. The emphasis will continue to fall on parents to protect their children from its hostile, exploitative elements rather than on creating a benevolent society that values its young and its own future. The first challenge is to recognize the denigration of parenthood as a form of juvenile ageism.

References

AP. (1998). Plan to sterilize woman is debated. *The New York Times*, September 25. https://www.nytimes.com/1988/09/25/us/plan-to-sterilize-woman-is-debated.html. Accessed 6 July 2018.

Bowman, C. D. (2012). *Culture of American families: A national survey*. Charlottesville: Institute for Advanced Studies in Culture, University of Virginia. http://iasc-culture.org/survey_archives/IASC_CAF_Survey.pdf. Accessed 6 July 2018.

Bryner, J. (2012, July 3). 5 Million babies born from IVF, other reproductive technologies. Live science. https://www.livescience.com/21355-5-million-babies-born-ivf-technologies.html. Accessed 6 July 2018.

Buder, L. (1988, May 26). Neglect cited in the deaths of 4 infants. *The New York Times*. https://www.nytimes.com/1988/05/26/nyregion/neglect-cited-in-the-deaths-of-4-infants.html. Accessed 6 July 2018.

Caplan, A. L. (1986). The ethics of in vitro fertilization. *Primary Care, 13*(2), 241–253. https://www.ncbi.nlm.nih.gov/pubmed/3636929. Accessed 6 July 2018.

Debolt, A. (2017, November 2). What happened to "Octomom" Nadya Suleman? Now in 2018. *Gazette Review.* https://gazettereview.com/2015/07/what-happened-to-octomom-nadya-suleman-new-updates-available/. Accessed 21 Sept 2018.

FreeChild Institute. https://freechild.org/. Accessed 6 July 2018.

Heide, K. M. (2013). *Understanding parricide: When sons and daughters kill parents.* New York: Oxford University Press.

HRW [Human Rights Watch]. (2010). Children's rights. https://www.hrw.org/topic/childrens-rights. Accessed 6 July 2018.

In Interest of JLW. (1981). https://law.justia.com/cases/wisconsin/supreme-court/1981/80-2191-9.html. Accessed 6 July 2018.

Jamison, P. (2013, August 19). Mom's words put trial on hold. *Tampa Bay Times.* http://www.tampabay.com/news/courts/criminal/opening-statements-expected-to-star-in-mctear-baby-death-case/2137162. Accessed 6 July 2018.

Jenny, C., & Isaac, R. (2006). The relation between child death and child maltreatment. *Archives of the Diseases of Children, 91*(3), 265–269.

Kelly, R. (2009, March 3). The real reasons octomom drives us crazy. *Newsweek.* http://www.newsweek.com/real-reasons-octomom-drives-us-crazy-76381. Accessed 6 July 2018.

Lee, F. R. (2009, November 20). To blacks, precious is 'demeaned' or 'angelic.' *The New York Times.* http://www.nytimes.com/2009/11/21/movies/21precious.html. Accessed 6 July 2018.

Lehr v. Robertson, 463 U.S. 248. (1983). https://supreme.justia.com/cases/federal/us/463/248/case.html. Accessed 6 July 2018.

Petit, M. (2011, October 17). Why child abuse is so acute in the US. *BBC News.* https://www.bbc.com/news/magazine-15193530. Accessed 6 July 2018.

Register Staff. (1993, May 18). Judge found Kimberly Martin innocent by reason of insanity and released her from custody. The *Des Moines Register*, p. 2.

Spargo, C. (2015, December 1). Florida woman who was switched at birth opens up about divorcing her biological parents, blowing her million-dollar settlement and being a mom to six children by four different fathers. *The Daily Mail.* http://www.dailymail.co.uk/news/article-3339699/Florida-woman-switched-birth-opens-divorcing-biological-parents-blowing-million-dollar-settlement-mom-six-children-four-different-fathers.html. Accessed 6 July 2018.

Strachan, R., Gowen, L. K., & Walker, J. S. (2009). *The 2009 Portland national youth summit report.* Portland: Research and Training Center on Family Support and Children's Mental Health, Portland State University. https://www.pathwaysrtc.pdx.edu/pdf/pbYouthSummitReport.pdf. Accessed 6 July 2018.

UNICEF. (n.d.). FACT SHEET: A summary of the rights under the Convention on the Rights of the Child. https://www.unicef.org/crc/files/Rights_overview.pdf. Accessed 6 July 2018.

UPI. (1994, July 26). Katie Beers' kidnapper gets 15 years. https://www.upi.com/Archives/1994/07/26/Katie-Beers-kidnapper-gets-15-years/8547775195200/ph. Accessed 6 July 2018.

Youth On Board. http://www.youthonboard.org/. Accessed 6 July 2018.

Chapter 9
The Devaluation of Parenthood

> *The proper officers will take the offspring of the good parents to the pen or fold, and there will deposit them with certain nurses who dwell in a separate quarter; but the offspring of the inferior, or of the better when they chance to be deformed, will be put away in some mysterious, unknown place, as they should be...*
>
> *They will provide for their nurture, and will bring the mothers to the fold when they are full of milk, taking the greatest possible care that no mother recognizes her own child...Care will also be taken that the process of suckling shall not be protracted too long; and the mothers will have no getting up at night or other trouble, but will hand all this sort of thing to the nurses and attendants.*
>
> Plato, The Republic, Book V (Plato n.d.)

Plato's perfect Republic was one in which children would be raised more efficiently by nurses than by parents who would be free to pursue their own interests. Plato's Republic had parents without parenthood.

Israeli Zionists in the early twentieth century thought the burden of childrearing and homemaking was the root cause of gender inequality. They emulated Plato's Utopian form of childrearing in their communes and tried to eliminate parenthood. They replaced marriage with cohabitation. A couple shared sleeping quarters but retained separate names and identities. Children were reared in community-run children's houses. Adults thought of kibbutz children as "joint social property" and were discouraged from developing close relationships with their offspring. Boys and girls were encouraged to think of the kibbutz itself as their parent. Thus freed from the domestic yoke, women engaged in productive work alongside men. Feminine clothes, cosmetics, jewelry, and hairstyles were rejected. In order to be equals, women had to look like men as well.

Similarly, royalty and the wealthy always have hired others to care for their children. This motif of delegating parenting now permeates the United States where the marketplace values only paid work, although it is encountering resistance from

© Springer Nature Switzerland AG 2019
J. C. Westman, *Dealing with Child Abuse and Neglect as Public Health Problems*, https://doi.org/10.1007/978-3-030-05897-5_9

those who prize raising their own children. This resistance by parents led ultimately to abolishing the separation of parents and children in kibbutzim. Today kibbutzim support parenthood highly with paid parental leave and work adjustments to accommodate parenting tasks and family living. The society that once attempted to abolish parenthood became a strong advocate of parenthood.

9.1   A Snapshot of American Parenthood

Parenthood generally is not accorded a high value in the United States. Having a baby is a status symbol … caring for one is not. Unlike other Western nations, the United States does not recognize the economic value of parenthood. Many parents are diverted from childrearing to paid employment either by choice or by necessity in welfare-to-work programs. Childcare is regarded as a marketable educational function rather than a fulfilling developmental experience for adults and children.

In her book *The Outsourced Self*, professor emeritus of sociology at the University of California-Berkeley Arlie Russell Hochschild (2012) points out that the rise of feminism coincided with a drastic lengthening of work hours and a steep decline in job security (Hochschild 2012). In the United States, those stressors have not been alleviated by social supports like paid family leave and universal childcare, at least not in comparison with most other Western nations. As a result too many family and community bonds are strained by anxious, overworked couples, too many family functions have been subcontracted, and too many children perceive themselves as burdens.

Our nation has viewed childrearing as a private matter unless it is terminated by death or abandonment or when parents damage their children by neglect or abuse. Otherwise our society has limited its role to public education. In many circles, parenthood has come to be regarded as an optional accessory rather than as a developmental stage in the life cycles of men and women. In his book *What to Expect When No One's Expecting*, Jonathan V. Last (2014) writes that pets now outnumber children four to one in American homes (Last 2014).

The disparagement of parenthood is felt particularly strongly by adults who place parenthood above employment away from home during their children's early lives. The term "working" women and men refers to people who are employed away from home and implies that homemaking is not work or at least is less important than paid work.

In addition, the economic benefit of the family has largely disappeared. Children are no longer economic assets and are costly liabilities instead. Most importantly, later chapters of this book will show how public policies and workplaces stack the odds against those who choose to raise our nation's children.

One result in all advanced nations has been a dramatic fall in birth rates—often too well below replacement rates—and rapidly aging populations. At the same time, the state of family life has become deeply problematic. High rates of divorce and out-of-wedlock births and increasing downward mobility of parents abound.

Marriage is being replaced by cohabitation. Virtually unheard of 30 years ago, homeless families are commonplace today.

It appears today that parenthood is not generally valued as a lifelong career in the United States. Due to the growth of Social Security, Medicare, and private pension options, support in old age no longer depends on an individual's decision to raise a family.

More adults are opting not to have children. Traditional marriage is being replaced by cohabitation. Meanwhile, the widening life options for both men and women in our society make nurturing the next generation a less attractive option. As it now stands, public policies and workplaces stack the odds against those who choose to raise children.

Still, people who bear the burdens of parenthood produce the vital human natural capital needed to keep our economic system going. We need to make major adjustments in our social policies in order to give parents a greater return from society for the costs of their investment in children. Because stable families produce productive citizens, our social policies should strengthen families. Because raising children is a public good, our Parent-Society Contract should support competent parenthood.

Few politicians want to tackle controversial issues, such as poverty, race, childrearing, family structure, and children's rights. Unfortunately, ensuring that newborns have competent parents evokes all of them and seems like a hopeless task.

Consequently, even though we know that incompetent parents harm their babies, families, and society, we act as if there is nothing we can do until their children are damaged by neglect or abuse. Meanwhile, we support them with both public and private funds.

We fail to protect our newborns because of deeply held beliefs beyond the prejudice that fuels juvenile ageism. The most important is our instinctive response to childbirth. Newborns are regarded as the personal property of their genetic mothers and fathers even if the latter are minors or developmentally disabled. The idea of separating babies from their parents is abhorrent.

We also believe that the experience of being a parent will bring out the best in anyone. The Horatio Alger theme is deeply embedded in our society. Certainly, adolescent parents have successfully raised their children and become productive citizens. Some even have become leaders and celebrities. We want to believe everyone can "make it" through diligent effort. We specifically hope that parenthood will give meaning and purpose in life to anyone.

Another deeply held belief involves "taking the consequences" of one's actions. The honorable response to childbirth under any circumstances may be marriage or at least for the unmarried mother and father to raise the baby. To this end, many families step forward to assist their adolescent parents or to raise their grandchildren themselves.

Moreover, our charitable impulse is to help the less fortunate. We feel obliged to minimize adversity for vulnerable parents and to improve their babies' lives by providing parenting education as well as childcare so adolescent parents can attend school.

We also do not trust public or private agencies to determine whether or not a parent is competent. That determination is made by a court acting upon a Child in Need of Protective Services petition.

In addition to creating the childcare industry as a capitalistic supplement to parenthood, our society is imbued with materialistic beliefs that encourage parents to seek alternatives to caring for their children. One widely held belief is that both parents should be employed away from home on a full-time basis in order to generate enough income to pay for high-quality childcare along with luxury goods and services.

Another belief is that commercially fostered trends of consumption reflect success and sophistication. Parents are attracted to professional expertise and novel technologies that free them from menial chores like childrearing. When you can pay someone else to do a tedious job better, why do it yourself? Even when childrearing appeals to adults, the lack of social support for a task regarded as "caretaking" or "caregiving" rather than as an interactive growth process for children and adults undermines its value.

Because children are the raison d'être of parenthood, anything that undermines parenthood detracts from children's developmental needs. Both obvious and subtle disparagement of parenthood adversely affects children.

9.2   Parenthood in Second Place

Our civilization's growing complexity brings competition among interests and activities. Childrearing is increasingly delegated to institutions, such as schools and childcare facilities. Rather than being the primary activity of adults, parenthood often is relegated to second place by necessity and by choice. Only one in three households in the United States has a child under the age of 18.

Because it is unpaid, parenthood does not have direct and immediate economic value while paying others to care for children does. Parents, therefore, seem to be more useful to society in the workforce where productivity can be valued in monetary terms. Hiring non-parents to care for children also creates jobs that increase the GDP. Still, childcare's financial value is comparatively low, and most is not of good quality.

A Gallup (2017) survey that found that employment away from home makes it easier for women to lead personally satisfying lives. It also makes raising children and maintaining a successful marriage more difficult when men do not value parenting and homemaking. Marriage and parenthood have been separated. Parenthood even seems to have become an obstacle to a successful marriage for some parents.

Jennifer Westfeldt's movie "Friends with Kids" questions why people need to experience romance with the same partner with whom they raise children. "Best intentions aside," Westfeldt says in a *New York Times* article, "having kids always changes your friendship ... in a way that I think is painful for both of you" (Kamminer 2012).

As with other civilizations, successive generations of Americans have been concerned about the deterioration of families as they adapt to new social conditions. In recent decades, consumerism has particularly affected family life. Following World War II, parents felt a strong commitment to give their children more material things than they had during their childhoods in the Great Depression. Overindulged children lost respect for parents and authority. The Vietnam War intensified the disillusionment of the young in their elders. Later decades were dominated by the Cold War and fear of nuclear attacks.

Now an anti-authority, postmodern philosophy permeates our society with its emphasis on self-assertive individualism. An ethos of avoiding discomfort and frustration has risen to the top. Both young and old adults can choose options that are "best for me." The pursuit of perfection further intensifies this ethos.

Henry Giroux (2007), professor of cultural studies at McMaster University, describes the growing commercialization of our everyday lives, the corporatization of education, the dismantling of welfare, the securitizing of public spaces, and the privatizing of public services. This trend has made it more difficult to develop family-friendly social policies that support parenthood.

9.3   Parenthood Is Not Seen as a Career

Most importantly, our society does not recognize parenthood as a career. It does not formally acknowledge that childrearing is skilled, hands-on work in which parents and children bond and grow together. It automatically awards full parental rights to any genetic parent regardless of age or ability until the child is damaged by the parent's neglect and/or abuse and parental rights are terminated by a court.

Nonetheless, parenthood is a lifelong career. Like any career, parenthood has its frustrations and rewards. Unlike any other career, it is based on affectionate attachment bonds. For most parents, parenthood is just as important as a paid career. This is especially evident during a person's later years. Louis Terman's Stanford study of eminent women and men found that, as they looked back on their lives, they valued family relationships over their professional careers (Terman 1925).

We need to face the implications of parenthood as a lifelong career. Family life is changing rapidly in the face of increasing maternal employment, father absence, and cultural diversity. Many parents need more than one income to make ends meet. In some families, parent-child roles are reversed. At the same time, children are being treated as commodities by reimbursed childcare systems. All of this takes place alongside increasing ambivalence about committed relationships and questions about who is the parent of a child conceived through IVF technologies.

Having "a parent" in itself means nothing to babies, children, and adolescents. Anyone past puberty can be a mother or a father, but to enter parenthood is to have a career with a lifelong commitment to a daughter or son. Parenthood means everything to babies, children, and adolescents. They need competent parents who can handle its responsibilities. Unfortunately, our society does not distinguish between merely being a mother or a father and motherhood and fatherhood. Consequently, it fails to ensure that our children have competent parents.

The extent to which parenthood can be demeaned inadvertently by child development professionals showed up in an article in ZERO TO THREE (2010), a professional journal devoted to early childhood that listed "the needs of infants." On the list is "Infants need a special someone." The word parent was replaced by special someone.

Contemporary ideas about childrearing emphasize talented and independent children. Annette Lareau (2002), a professor of sociology at the University of Maryland, notes that many upper-middle-class parents provide learning experiences for their children at an exhausting pace. In contrast, lower-middle-class parents seem to believe that adulthood will come soon enough and that children should be left alone to create their own play. These children seem more relaxed and vibrant and appear to enjoy more intimate contact with their extended families. Lareau commented:

> Whining, which was pervasive in middle-class homes, was rare in working-class homes. Middle-class adolescents feel entitled to individual treatment... Working-class adolescents feel constrained....

The rewards of parenthood are easily obscured for contemporary parents who have not discovered the satisfactions and pleasures of parenthood. Instead, they try to "have it all now" for themselves and their children.

Plato's idea of raising children away from their parents was not realized in ancient Greece. It failed in all subsequent childrearing experiments from the Israeli kibbutzim to the People's Republic of China. Even the wealthy who delegate childrearing often do not have rewarding family relationships. Still Plato's idea has resonance in the United States.

Moreover, our social values do not formally articulate parenthood standards except for adoptive and foster parents. However, our cultural values do hold expectations for people who give birth to a child. The vast majority of children are raised by parents who fulfill these cultural expectations by building and maintaining parent-child bonds, but an increasing number are not. Pediatrician T. Berry Brazelton and child psychiatrist Stanley Greenspan (2002) suggested in their book *The Irreducible Needs of Children* that this underlies the general fragility of relationships in our society. Adults who did not have caring, intimate relationships with their parents find sustaining committed relationships, including with spouses and offspring, difficult.

Because committed relationships are vital to our society's integrity and prosperity, we must articulate our cultural expectations of parenthood, the source of committed relationships. Implicit cultural expectations include children's moral right to competent parents and their obligation to respect and cooperate with their parents. These cultural expectations have evolved into legal expectations codified in child abuse and neglect statutes. Because our society has not sufficiently valued parenthood, courts are increasingly involved in articulating our cultural expectations of parenthood.

9.4 The Role of Courts in Defining Parenthood

Courts no longer hold that the human right to procreate also accords ownership of the child. When family matters are adjudicated, a variety of case and common law precedents define our expectations of parents based on our cultural values. Child abuse and neglect cases as well as divorce custody laws articulate these expectations.

In family courts, our cultural expectations of parenthood are to:

- Provide a home that legitimizes a child's identity in a community
- Provide sufficient income for a child's clothing, shelter, education, health care, and social and recreational activities
- Provide the love, security, and emotional support necessary for healthy development
- Foster intellectual, social, and moral development
- Socialize the child by setting limits and encouraging civil behavior
- Protect the child from physical, emotional, and social harm
- Maintain stable family interactions through communication, problem solving, and responses to individual needs

When we look at these expectations, we can see that we really do rely on parents to instill cultural values so that children will become responsible citizens. The need to explicitly recognize the essential role of parenthood and to support parents in childrearing becomes obvious. Parental incompetence at any point in a child's development can have unintended long-term consequences.

9.4.1 Defining Parental Competence

Because we all fall short of our idealized expectations, most parents tend to doubt their competence. An initial reaction to any discussion of competence might be to judge oneself as less than competent. This overreaction creates a reluctance to deal with actual parental incompetence since doing so might involve judging all parents. In fact, the vast majority of parents are competent.

Competent parents quite simply are committed to parenthood. Their behavior shows that they care about their children. They restrain themselves from harming them. They do not neglect or abuse their children in a legal sense. The definition of competent parents flows from our cultural expectations: competent parents are capable of assuming responsibility for their own lives, sacrificing some of their interests for their children, providing limits for their children's behavior, and giving their children hope for the future. They also have access to essential economic and educational resources. When necessary, society has an obligation to provide access to these resources. Just as there are dietary elements essential for physical growth, there are essential experiences for healthy personality growth. Children must learn to delay gratification, tolerate frustration, work productively, and avoid harming others.

Young people acquire the values and skills essential for success through parents who possess these qualities. This does not mean that competent parents are social conformists who raise conforming children to become conforming adults. Our democratic republic depends as much upon parents who initiate changes. Our way of life depends upon diversity in opinions and lifestyles.

Most importantly, wealth does not ensure parental competence nor does poverty ensure parental incompetence. The empirical fact is that children raised by competent parents — including the poor and the physically handicapped — seldom become criminals or welfare dependent.

9.4.2   Defining Parental Incompetence

A child's congenital handicaps and the lack of socioeconomic resources can make parenthood stressful for even the most competent adults. Incompetent parents, on the other hand, cannot take responsibility for their own lives, much less for their children's. In legal terms, they are "unfit." Most minimize or deny their incompetence. Their lack of skills can stem from immaturity or from personality, developmental and mental disorders, or addictions. Even with support and treatment, many are unable to change soon enough to raise their own children.

Because incompetent parents have difficulty controlling their impulses, they are vulnerable to substance abuse and alcoholism. They are insensitive to the needs of others and are unreliable. They do not form stable attachment bonds with their children. They alternately neglect or overreact to their children's behavior with unpredictable and inconsistent cycles of indifference, idle threats, and severe punishment. They have difficulty restraining themselves from harming their children. Their children are confused when what happens to them bears little relationship to what they do. The parents' erratic behaviors result in inconsistent childrearing practices. As a result, the children of incompetent parents are insensitive to the needs of others and behave unpredictably. These children often become adults who do not control their impulses and who do not care how their behavior affects other people.

Incompetent parents can be detected without subtle techniques or tests. No unbiased, fully informed person would have any difficulty identifying them. A conservative look at child neglect and abuse reports reveals that about 4% of all parents are incompetent according to the above definition. This represents 8% of one-parent and 3% of two-parent homes. Although small in percentage, the number is significant…6.6 million. At least twice as many parents have not yet been adjudicated as abusive or neglectful (CDC 2014).

Most people do not appreciate the impact this comparatively small number of parents has on our society until the number of incompetent parents is multiplied by the number of children they produce. One in four children (11 million) have been damaged by abuse and/or neglect. A larger number have had their lives impaired enough to create later adverse effects on their own offspring.

Neglect by incompetent parents is more harmful than physical abuse. It eliminates any opportunity to develop the social skills children need to become responsible human beings. In contrast, children who are abused but not neglected may be able to relate to other people. In that way, they may be able to acquire the social skills needed for productive citizenship.

Damage caused by parental neglect is clear in developmentally delayed babies whose "failure to thrive" stems from the lack of attachment bonds. These babies do not feed properly and suffer severe enough delays in their physical, social, and cognitive development to result in death.

The lack of prevention programs and the inability of child welfare services to therapeutically intervene with incompetent parents create situations our society no longer should tolerate. The following is a typical case example:

Mary was born to a sixteen-year-old alcoholic mother, who subsisted on Aid to the Families of Dependent Children and divorced twice before Mary was first brought to the attention of child welfare services at the age of 3 because of repeated allegations of parental neglect.

At the age of 9, Mary began to be sexually abused by an older brother. When she was 10, she was placed in a special class for the emotionally disturbed. When 13, she was brought to juvenile court because of alcohol and substance abuse and a year later placed in a county juvenile home. Her destructive behavior led to subsequent placement in two adolescent treatment centers.

When 15, Mary was sent to a state correctional facility and thereafter to a state mental hospital. After her release at 18, her first child was born. She subsequently was married and divorced three times. Her second child was born when she was 20. When her children were 2 and 4 years old, child welfare services intervened and placed the children in foster homes. Mary entered two alcohol and substance abuse treatment centers and did not complete treatment. She was arrested several times for drinking while driving, once in a near-fatal accident and later for the sale of illegal drugs. She sought and obtained the return of her children after serving three months in jail. Within two months Mary resumed drinking. Her children were placed again in foster care at the ages of 4 and 6. By that time their behavior problems necessitated psychiatric treatment.

When 25, Mary was sentenced to prison because of drug dealing. Her parental rights were finally terminated, and her children were placed in adoptive homes where they continued in psychiatric treatment and special education.

We must recognize that not all people who conceive and give birth are competent parents. Identifying incompetent parents before they damage their children must be a high priority. Those who cannot be competent parents need relief from the responsibilities of parenthood through expeditious termination of their parental rights followed by adoption.

9.5   The Roles of Parenthood

Our society has a vital interest in ensuring that all children have competent parents. The two roles of parenthood, motherhood and fatherhood, should be thoroughly understood as part of this process.

9.5.1   Motherhood

A society's attitude toward motherhood is influenced by its attitude toward children. One consequence of juvenile ageism fully described in succeeding chapters is the devaluation of motherhood and of caring for the young.

Welfare-to-work policies require mothers to take low-paying jobs even though maternal care during the 1st year is less costly than publicly funded childcare. Employment, therefore, is cast as more important than parenting. This is true even though parenting can reduce public expenditures and is in the interests of babies and mothers. More broadly, motherhood brings one of the most difficult decisions in a woman's life…stay at home, pursue a career, or do both?

Often motherhood is seen as something that interferes with paid careers. In her book *Get to Work*, Linda Hirshman, an emeritus professor of women's studies at Brandeis University, believes childrearing is not fulfilling for educated women. She is concerned about the current trend in which women are leaving the workforce to become full-time mothers.

Hirshman believes that the family with its repetitious, socially invisible tasks is a necessary social institution but that it does not allow women to flourish. Careers in business or government, after all, offer money and professional advancement as markers of success. Hirshman suggests that women devote their first few years after college to preparation for paid work. She wrote:

> Expensively educated mothers who stay at home are leading lesser lives. They bear the burden of work associated with lower social classes—housekeeping and childcare. (Hirshman 2006)

According to Leslie Bennetts, journalist and author, employed mothers are best for children (Mead 2006). They exemplify resourcefulness and independence, and they demonstrate the virtue of engaging in work one loves. She suggests that women lose their humanity if they do not fulfill themselves through paid careers. In her book *The Conflict*, Elizabeth Badinter (2012) holds that an exalted view of motherhood can have the effect of controlling women and seeking to reconcile them to a lack of independence and frustrating their individual talents and ambitions (Badinter 2012). In contrast, novelist Lisa Jackson said that empowering yourself does not have to mean rejecting motherhood or eliminating the nurturing or feminine aspects of who you are (Slaughter 2012).

The demeaning of motherhood also is reflected in the dramatic changes in women's labor force patterns over the last 20 years. Many more mothers now work full or part time. The wage gap between men and women has narrowed but persists. According to the 2017 Bureau of Labor Statistics, the median weekly wage for men was $915 and for women $749 (Bureau of Labor Statistics 2018). Mothers earned about $1.50 an hour less than childless women. If they continue to be largely responsible for childrearing, mothers will not catch up. Since most women have children, this penalty continues to contribute to workplace inequality.

Still, the Barnard College Parenting Young Children Study revealed that most mothers felt overwhelmed by the conflicting demands of raising children and employed careers but desired to do both well (Klein et al. 2006). When one had to give, most mothers were not willing to sacrifice the interests of their families.

In their book *Mass Career Customization*, Cathleen Benko and Ann Weisberg (2007) show how today's career path no longer means a straight march up the corporate ladder but rather a combination of climbs, lateral moves, and planned descents. According to Sylvia Ann Hewlett of the Center for Work-Life Policy, 37% of all professional women leave employment at some point to rear children (Hewlett and Luce 2005). Even more have flexible schedules, but only 40% of those who return to employment find full-time jobs. Even then, employment usually comes with a loss of earnings. This pattern has been exaggerated by the recession that began in 2008.

9.5.2   Fatherhood

The need to establish paternity for newborns underscores the vulnerability of fatherhood. In our society, almost 40% of all babies are born to unmarried mothers. To try to ensure that the babies obtain the support of both parents, federal policies encourage establishing paternity as soon as possible. This increases the likelihood that the baby will have a lasting relationship with the father and that child support will be paid. Different jurisdictions vary widely in rates of establishing paternity and in child support awards.

The form fatherhood takes also varies more widely than motherhood. Fathers are involved with their children in three ways:

- Living with their children
- Visitation with their children
- Responsibility for their children's support without a relationship

A University of Michigan Institute of Social Research study revealed that at some point in their lives, half of all children don't live with their biological fathers (Hartnett et al. 2016). During a 30-year period, 28% of the men who lived with the mothers at the time the children were born moved away. Men who cohabited with the mothers were more than twice as likely to live away from the children as married men. Forty-one percent of black fathers do not live with their children compared to 24% of white fathers.

The casual, unrealistic attitudes fathers can hold toward conceiving children is revealed by two young fathers:

- Twenty-year-old Anthony explained, "I'll use a condom with other girls, but not with my special girlfriend. Pregnancy, like, is for her. Still marriage is a big step. I might have a baby with her, but I haven't found Miss Right yet."
- Nineteen-year-old Carmelo sold drugs so that his 2-year-old daughter could have "everything I wanted her to have. I felt like if I had a kid, it would settle me down." He took a GED course for a few months and spent less time hanging out

with his friends. His girlfriend Shana thought getting pregnant would force Carmelo to stay around. She ended up on welfare after Carmelo left her.

9.6   Can Parenthood Be Valued Again in the United States?

Social progressives look to Scandinavia as a model for child wellbeing. If the United States adopted Sweden's or Norway's generous family benefits, they argue, we too could achieve low rates of child poverty, adolescent pregnancy, and single parenthood. Social conservatives point to Sweden as a cautionary example of how generous social welfare policies can weaken marriage and the family.

Neither side tells the whole story. Scandinavian cultures are child-friendly in the sense that children have basic rights. Their cultures stress an individual's responsibility to the common good of society in contrast with the American emphasis on individualism and on adult rights that tend to regard children as the property of their parents.

Child poverty barely exists in Sweden, and adolescent birth rates are very low. Few babies are in childcare because mothers have 1 year of paid family leave following childbirth. The Swedish marriage rate is one of the lowest in the world, while divorce rates continue to rise. Sweden leads the Western nations in cohabitation. Breakups for these couples occur twice as frequently as in marriage.

The Swedish approach includes policies that many social conservatives would embrace such as strict limits on abortion, a 6-month waiting period before divorce, a ban on IVF procedures for single women and anonymity for sperm donors. Still, the United States and Sweden are among the developed nations with the lowest percentage of children growing up with both genetic parents.

Despite these commonalities, the two societies are very different. Sweden is communitarian, comparatively ethnically homogeneous, socially cohesive, and resolutely secular. America is individualistic, ethnically diverse, and possibly strongly religious. Though Scandinavian family policies might be models for a more child-friendly society, we cannot simply adopt their social policies and achieve the same results. The common good is a paramount value in their culture; individualism is paramount in the United States.

9.7   Where Does This Leave Us?

In the United States, anyone past puberty can be a parent, but parenthood is a life-long commitment to a son or a daughter. Only competent adults can handle its responsibilities. Work is defined in our capitalistic economy as a paid activity. Unpaid activities like childrearing are not regarded as work. This obscures the fact that childrearing has immense financial value. In the long run, parenthood is more important for our society's prosperity than paid vocations. Although not recognized as such, parenthood is the career that benefits everyone whether it is in one-parent or two-parent homes.

9.7.1   Statistics

According to the Pew Research Center, in 2017, 50% of all adults in the United States were married (Parker and Stepler 2017). Many who marry are not interested in parenthood. Fortunately, neither the survival of the species nor individual fulfillment depends upon every person becoming a parent. Fewer families today fit the traditional image of two married parents living with their genetic children. In 2014:

- Of all households, 33% included children.
- Of households including children, 61% consisted of married couples, 26% consisted of mother only homes, 7% consisted of cohabiting couples, and 6% father only homes.
- Twenty-one percent of married couples and 59% of unmarried couples had children from more than one relationship.

According to the 2017 US Census Bureau data, out of about 12 million single-parent families with children under the age of 18, more than 80% were headed by single mothers (US Census 2018).

Marica Carlson and Paula England (2011) point out in their book *Changing Families* in an Unequal Society that, except for college-educated Americans, marriage continues to be less appealing. Individuals are marrying later and cohabiting more often. This trend contributes to an increasing gap in wellbeing between college-graduate married families and less-educated unmarried families.

In 2016, families maintained by women were less likely to have an employed member (76.6%) than families maintained by men (83.6%) or married-couple families (81.1%). Among married-couple families, both the husband and wife were employed in 48% of families, in 19.5% of married-couple families only the husband was employed, and in 7.1% only the wife was employed (US Bureau of Labor Statistics 2018). In 2016, 40% of all births were to unmarried girls and women (20% one-parent and 20% cohabiting) with 60% of births occurring with married couples (CDC n.d.).

9.7.2   Attitudes

A 2007 Pew survey found that Americans of all ages believed the link between marriage and parenthood had weakened (Pew Research Center 2007). Just 41% of Americans said children are "very important" to a successful marriage, down from 65% in 1990. Children have fallen to eighth out of nine things people associate with successful marriages, well behind "sharing household chores, good housing, adequate income, happy sexual relationship, and faithfulness."

On the other hand, the Michigan Study of Adolescent Life Transitions revealed that despite greater acceptance of divorce, premarital sex, and non-marital cohabitation since the 1960s, positive attitudes toward marriage and parenthood remain strong among high school seniors (MSALT 2015). Eighty-eight percent of male and 83% of female seniors said it was quite or extremely important to have a good marriage and family life.

In 2003, 75% of college freshmen named raising a family as an important life goal, up from 59% in 1977. However, only 1 in 1000 chose full-time homemaker as their probable career. Almost 70% of adolescent boys and 54% of girls agreed it is better for a person to get married than to go through life being single. They also felt that divorce is not the best solution to marital problems.

A Child Trends survey found that adolescents knew that a healthy relationship should be marked by respect, honesty, fidelity, good communication, and the absence of violence (Guzman et al. 2009). At the same time, many expressed pessimism about their chances of ever experiencing that type of relationship. Nor did they know many adults whose romantic relationships were worthy of emulation.

In a National Health and Social Life Survey, men expressed a desire to marry but were in no hurry to do so because they (Wilcox and Wolfinger 2017):

- Can get sex without marriage more easily than in the past
- Can have a companion by cohabiting rather than marrying
- Want to avoid divorce and its financial risks
- Are waiting for the perfect soul mate
- Face few social pressures to marry
- Are reluctant to marry a woman who already has children
- Want to own a house before marrying

More than half of the young men surveyed reported changing jobs and a variety of living arrangements including returning to their parents' homes. Male friends were their stable attachments.

9.8 Adolescent Parenthood and Marriage

Despite a nearly one-third decline over the past decade in adolescent pregnancy and birth rates in the United States according to Power to Decide, the campaign to prevent unplanned pregnancy (Power to Decide 2018):

- Sixty percent of all girls aged 15 through 17 and 73% of ages 18–19 approve of unwed childbearing.
- Half of all first unwed births are to adolescents.
- Within 1 year of childbirth, 8% of adolescent mothers marry the genetic fathers.
- Only 30% of adolescent mothers who do marry are still in that marriage at the age of 40.

9.9 Cohabitation

Over the years, marriage has lost ground as the context for childrearing and become more exclusively an intimate relationship between adults. This transition has come through piecemeal changes with little consideration of the social consequences of a weaker connection between marriage and childrearing.

The ethos of individualism has made unmarried cohabitation the lifestyle of choice for many young people. Formerly referred to as "shacking up" or "living in sin," cohabitation has become common. In 1994, two-thirds of respondents under the age of 30 in the National Survey of Families and Households felt that unmarried sex, cohabitation, and unmarried births were socially acceptable (RWJF 2018). In 2001, 88% of young men and 93% of young women agreed that it is usually a good idea for a couple to live together before getting married. More than 50% of boys and girls now believe that having a child out of wedlock is an acceptable lifestyle that does not affect anyone else. In 2006–2008, 58% of women ages 19–44 had cohabited. Cohabitation apparently functions as a substitute for being single rather than as a substitute for marriage or parenthood.

A 2012 analysis of the Princeton Fragile Families and Child Wellbeing Study suggests there are only slight negative implications for children raised in stable two-genetic-parent cohabiting families compared to stable two-genetic-married-parent families (Fragile Families 2018). The difference appears to be largely due to differences in the backgrounds of parents who choose cohabitation over marriage. Once these personal factors are taken into account, children of both kinds of stable parental relationships appear similar in terms of behavior problems. Children of cohabiting genetic parents who marry after childbirth appear no better off than the children of cohabiting genetic parents who remain unmarried as long as the relationship of the latter is stable.

On the one hand, these findings might indicate that marital unions are no more beneficial to children than cohabiting unions of biological parents as long as the relationship remains stable. On the other hand, marriages are more stable than cohabiting relationships. In cohabiting families, children move in and out of different family arrangements more often. The empirical fact is that cohabitation preceding marriage does not ensure a stable marriage later on.

9.10 Single-Parent Homes

Although it might not seem so at first, the words used to describe contemporary families are important. Two-parent homes occur with and without marriage. When one parent is a nonresident, a family can be located in two homes. When a mother and father live separately, single-parent family does not accurately define the situation since one-parent homes can serve a two-parent family because the other parent lives elsewhere. Each can be with or without genetic parents. No wonder the word family confuses children, parents, and researchers.

When parenthood generally referred to married adults, single parenthood resulted from the death or divorce of a parent. Adolescent parenthood was not formally recognized. In recent decades, personal choice has replaced cultural traditions in defining parenthood. Married parents now feel less obliged to stay together for the sake of their children. Separation usually is stressful for children but so is relentless conflict that is not resolved by counseling.

Currently, most parents are not single by death or divorce. According to the National Survey of Family Growth, the number of babies born to unwed women in their 30s and 40s rose by 290% from 1980 to 2002. Non-marital births and birth rates have declined 7% and 14%, respectively, since peaking in the late 2000s. About 40% of U.S. births were to unmarried women in each year from 2007 to 2013 (CDC 2014). At some point in their lives, almost half of all children born in the United States will have lived in one-parent homes, primarily headed by women. More than half of those will live in poverty for a time and will continue the cycle of family disadvantage.

The organization Single Mothers by Choice is a support network for single women who have children without a relationship with a man (Single Mothers By Choice n.d.). Three-quarters conceived with donor sperm. Their members typically are career women in their 30s or 40s who decided to give birth or adopt knowing they would be their child's sole parent. Biological pressure meant they could no longer wait for marriage before starting a family. They became pregnant accidentally or from donor insemination, or they adopted a child. They seek men as out-of-home "social capital" (father figures) for their children.

Whether parents in the United States are married, cohabiting or raising children without a partner, they are more likely to change living arrangements than parents in the rest of the Western world.

Over the past 40 years, the greater financial independence of women contributed to the increase in one-parent homes facilitated by (1) the decline in family size, (2) the increase in divorce rates, (3) expansion of the service sector where most women are employed, (4) an increase in women's earnings, and (5) civil rights legislation. These trends improved women's occupations as well as their earnings.

National social policies influence the wellbeing of children in one-parent homes. Countries with low single-mother poverty rates have a combination of child allowances, guaranteed child support, unemployment assistance, and housing allowances for low-income families that benefit both one- and two-parent homes.

Without an impossible experiment where children are randomly assigned to different kinds of families, we do not know how children in one-parent homes would have fared if they had lived with two genetic parents. Most one-parent homes raise their children successfully; however, their children do have more problems than those raised in two-parent homes.

The reason a home has only one parent is important. Kevin Lang, professor of economics at Boston University, and Jay Zagorsky, professor of economics at Ohio State University, found little evidence that the death of a parent affects children's economic wellbeing in adulthood (Lang and Zagorsky 2001). However, a mother's death might reduce a girl's cognitive performance, while a father's death might lower a son's chances of marriage.

Although children of divorced parents have more adjustment problems than children of parents who never divorced, the divorce itself might not be the cause. Many of the problems seen in children of divorce can be accounted for by experiences in earlier years, such as marital conflict, violence, and inadequate parenting.

9.11 Impact on Children

The Princeton Fragile Families Project has established the fact that one-parent homes are associated with a host of problems (Fragile Families 2018). This especially is true if the parents are uneducated and unemployed. Poverty forces mothers to rear children in neighborhoods with high rates of unemployment, school dropouts, adolescent pregnancy, and crime.

Children who live in one-parent homes have lower academic achievement than those in two-parent homes. Controlling for age, gender, and grade level, secondary school students living in one-parent homes score lower on mathematics and science tests than those in two-married-parent homes. Children in stepparent homes score somewhat higher than one-parent homes, but children living with two genetic parents score the highest. Those who live with their mother and an unmarried, non-genetic, cohabitating partner score the lowest.

Children living with both genetic parents remain in school longer than children in one-parent homes. High school graduation rates were 90% for those in two genetic-parent homes, 75% for those in divorced-mother homes, and 69% for those in unwed-mother homes.

Children with absent fathers are more likely to drop out of school than children who live with their fathers. Seventy-one percent of children who lived with two genetic parents go to college compared to 50% of children living only with their mothers. Each additional year spent with a single mother reduces a child's educational attainment by half a year, as does time spent in stepparent families.

Some of the impacts are much riskier. Children who spend part of their childhood in a single-mother home are twice as likely to have sex at an early age as children who live with both genetic parents. Daughters from single-mother homes also begin marital and non-marital childbearing at a younger age.

Whereas girls from two-parent homes have a 6% chance of having a child outside marriage by the age of 20, chances for girls from divorced single-mother and unwed families are 11% and 14%, respectively. Girls in stepfamilies have a 16% chance of unwed childbirth.

Growing up in a single-mother home is strongly linked to income later in life. Timothy Biblarz and Adrian Raftery reported in their article Family Structure, Educational Attainment, and Socioeconomic Success that children from high occupational status homes were less likely to end up in high-status occupations if they came from a single-mother home (Biblartz and Faferty 1999). Sara McLanahan and Gary Sandefur reported in their book *Growing Up with a Single Parent* that adults from single-mother homes were more likely to be unemployed and on welfare than those from two-parent homes (McLanahan and Sandefur 1997; Demo 1996).

9.12   Father's Absence

A meta-analysis of the literature on father absence by the Princeton Center for Research on Child Wellbeing found lower levels of behavioral problems in adolescents living with married genetic parents than with all other family styles (Harper and McLanahan n.d.).

While over 90% of all American children live with their genetic mothers at some time, only about 50% spend at least part of their lives with their genetic fathers. Children who do not live with their genetic fathers often are disadvantaged by low income and poor relationships between and with their parents.

The annual expenditures made by the federal government to support father-absent homes total $100 billion a year. These expenditures include 13 means tested benefit programs and child support enforcement.

Growing up without two parents who support each other is a significant contributor to drug abuse and delinquency. This is especially true when accompanied by poverty. When fathers are absent, children might be less well monitored because their mothers work longer hours.

Children who live apart from their genetic fathers are more likely to use illegal substances and to be arrested. Children below the age of 15 who live in a household without a father are 70% more likely to commit crimes and 28% more likely to use marijuana than children who live with both genetic parents. Children living apart from their genetic fathers are 19% more likely to smoke cigarettes than others.

Children with behavior problems might push fathers away, while well-behaved children might draw them in, but the behavior of parents has a greater effect on children than the behavior of children has on parents. Even if fathers become more involved, their children's behavioral problems might not decrease.

When nonresident fathers maintain a high-quality relationship with their children, some of the negative consequences of their absence can be attenuated. Currently, there is interest in using social policies to strengthen father-family involvement, such as through counseling, mentoring, marriage education, and enhancing relationship and parenting skills and by fostering economic stability.

9.12.1   Impact on Girls

When fathers are absent, girls have few opportunities to learn how to relate to males. A father-daughter relationship sets the stage for her romantic choices, shapes her sexuality, and influences her sense of herself as a woman. Developing an affectionate attachment with her father is important as a girl works through the Electra complex in which she fantasies marrying her father and displacing her mother. By working through this process, she comes to terms with the fantasy's impracticality.

Without a father's dependable involvement in her life, a girl lacks a model of adult male-female relationships as well as a tangible model of healthy masculinity.

Daughters need father figures who can be counted on at or away from home. When they do not receive the attention and affection they desire from their fathers, they might seek it elsewhere. This quest leads to early and unstable relationships. The situation is compounded when mothers are depressed. The following was written by 13-year-old Crystal for the National Center for Fathering (2009):

> I see my father a lot in my dreams but never does he turn around. I call for him, but he's just walking away. Every time I blow out the candles on my birthday cake, I wish that stranger would turn around and look at me. Maybe if he saw all the pain and suffering from living without him in my eyes, he would become a part of my life.

At the same time, if the relationship between father and daughter is too intense, a father might become the admired male in her life. She fulfills the Electra fantasy by becoming his primary love. When an incestuous relationship actually occurs, a girl suffers the consequences of sexual abuse. Her later life as a wife and a mother is adversely affected.

Children raised without a biological father have earlier average ages of first sexual intercourse than children raised in households where the father is present (Mendle et al. 2009).

Both girls and boys might feel their fathers left their home because they did not love them. One son put it this way: "A dad wouldn't leave a good kid, so it must have been my fault."

9.12.2 Impact on Boys

Boys usually first identify with their mothers. When a father is not available, boys have difficulty resolving the Oedipal complex in which they fantasize marrying their mothers and displacing the fathers. They cannot readily shift their identification from mother to father. This can lead to guilt over their unresolved fantasies. Repression of their masculinity might result. They can have difficulty developing and sustaining self-respect, forming lasting emotional attachments, recognizing their feelings, and expressing themselves later with adult partners and their own children.

Boys also might focus on their fathers' faults as a way to deny their need for a father. One boy said he could prove he did not need his father. Before taking any action, he imagined what his father would do and did the opposite. He claimed, "I don't need anyone." In contrast, another boy on the verge of tears described his feelings about his absent father:

> If my dad was still around, I wouldn't do so much dumb stuff. I'm pretty sure I'd be a good student. I'd have friends that were better for me. When I turn into a dad, I'm going to be different from my dad.

On the other hand, boys can contradict the stereotype that a boy suffers without a man in the home by growing into successful men. Journalist Peggy Drexler (2005) interviewed a group of what she called "maverick moms," relatively affluent and highly educated lesbians and single mothers by choice who were raising sons in San Francisco. The boys were socially savvy and generous while also being passionate about sports and roughhousing. Still, the families she interviewed were on society's fringes. Drexler viewed those maverick moms as pioneers of a new parenting style. They reject social judgments about family structure and gender stereotypes and stress communication, community, and love.

9.12.3   Perspectives on Fathers

In their own minds, no boy or girl is without a dad. In the absence of fathers, they make up their own images. Even when disappointed or abused by their fathers, children may create images of loving fathers in order to bolster their own self-respect. Eleanor Roosevelt wrote about her love for her father in spite of his alcoholism and abandonment of her (Roosevelt 2002).

When fathers are rarely or never seen, children depend on their mothers or other relatives for information about them. If a mother speaks about an absent father realistically, a child is more likely to develop a positive image in spite of the father's failings. She might despise him, but, if his problems can be understood, a child can develop a realistic image. This also applies to absent mothers.

Absent fathers miss an important developmental experience. Engaged fatherhood promotes a man's ability to understand himself, to understand others, and to integrate his feelings in intimate relationships with family members. Fathers are more likely to give back to their communities than childless men.

Most absent fathers pay support and are in touch with their children. Some might feel that mothers claim support for themselves rather than the children. If mothers fail to accept or sustain father-child relationships, the fathers can feel frustrated and victimized.

When fathers see themselves as victims whose rights are ignored, they become resistant and disengaged. Nonpayment of child support can be seen as a father's defiance or as a moral failing. Divorced, noncustodial "deadbeat fathers" tend to agree that "bad" fathers exist, but that applies to others not themselves. They accept an obligation to contribute to their children's support but often deem the amount or its terms unfair.

9.13   Whither Parenthood?

In recent decades, parenthood has been increasingly defined by choice. Single parenthood, cohabitation, divorce, gay-lesbian relationships, and remarriage have created a variety of family lifestyles. Strong currents operate against both our cultural values and the scientific knowledge that affirm children's need for the love and nurturing of both of their parents. As the significance of marriage has declined, single parenthood by choice or necessity has become common.

Marriage has supported middle-class foresight, planning, and self-sufficiency. It has organized women and men around nurturing children's cognitive, emotional, and physical development. Now, it separates successful middle-class children with both parents from their less-parented, underachieving lower-class peers. The United States appears to be moving toward a de facto hereditary caste society based on family structure.

We need to make major adjustments in our social contract with them to give parents a greater return for their investment in children. Because stable families produce productive citizens, our social contract should strengthen families. Because raising children is a public good, our Parent-Society Contract should support parenthood.

Children prick our consciences. They painfully remind us that we are flawed models, yet they also evoke our highest ideals. Although conflicts between the interests of older and younger generations are inevitable, the American cultural tradition is to promote competent parenthood. Still, there is a hidden barrier to achieving this goal—juvenile ageism that obscures the rights and needs of children, especially newborn babies.

References

Badinter, E. (2012). *The conflict: How modern motherhood undermines the status of women.* New York: Metropolitan Books.

Benko, C., & Weisberg, A. (2007). *Mass career customization: Aligning the workplace with today's non-traditional workforce.* Oakland: Deloitte Development LLC.

Biblarz, T. J., & Raftery, A. E. (1999). Family structure, educational attainment, and socioeconomic success: Rethinking the "pathology of matriarchy". *American Journal of Sociology, 105*(2), 321–365. http://www.jstor.org/stable/10.1086/210314?seq=1#page_scan_tab_contents. Accessed 6 July 2018.

Bureau of Labor Statistics. (2018, April 13). Usual weekly earnings summary, economic news release. https://www.bls.gov/news.release/wkyeng.nr0.htm. Accessed 6 July 2018.

Carlson, M. J., & England, P. (Eds.). (2011). *Social class and changing families in an unequal America.* Stanford: Stanford University Press.

CDC [Centers for Disease Control and Prevention]. (2014). Recent declines in nonmarital childbearing in the United States. NCHS Data Brief No. 162, August 2014. https://www.cdc.gov/nchs/data/databriefs/db162.htm. Accessed 6 July 2018.

CDC [Centers for Disease Control and Prevention]. (n.d.). National Center for Health Statistics. Percentage of births to unmarried mothers by state. https://www.cdc.gov/nchs/pressroom/sosmap/unmarried/unmarried.htm. Accessed 6 July 2018.

Demo, D. H. (1996). Review of *growing up with a single parent: What hurts, what helps* by Sara McLanahan and Gary Sandefur. Family Relations, *45,* 244. https://libres.uncg.edu/ir/uncg/f/D_Demo_Review_1996.pdf. Accessed 6 July 2018.

Drexler, P. (2005). Truth vs. myth … today's maverick moms are raising tomorrow's exceptional men! *Single Mother, 84*(Fall/Winter), 10. 11, 15. http://www.peggydrexler.com/articles/PeggyDrexler3.2.06.pdf. Accessed 6 July 2018.

Fragile Families and Child Well-Being Study. (2018). Princeton University. https://fragilefamilies.princeton.edu/documentation. Accessed 6 July 2018.

Gallup. (2017). State of the American workplace, p. 43. https://qualityincentivecompany.com/wp-content/uploads/2017/02/SOAW-2017.pdf. Accessed 6 July 2018.

Giroux, H. A. (2007). *Democracy's promise and the politics of worldliness in the age of terror.* CLCWeb: Comparative Literature and Culture 9.1. https://docs.lib.purdue.edu/cgi/viewcontent.cgi?article=1016&context=clcweb. Accessed 6 July 2018.

Guzman, L., Ikramullah, E., et al. (2009). *Telling it like it is: Teen perspectives on romantic relationships.* Washington, DC: Child Trends Research Brief. Publication #2009-44. https://www.childtrends.org/wp-content/uploads/2009/10/Child_Trends-2009_11_05_RB_TeenRelation.pdf. Accessed 6 July 2018.

Harper, C. C., & McLanahan, S. S. (n.d.). Father absence and youth incarceration. Center for Research on Child Wellbeing Working Paper #99-03. http://www.sharedparentinginc.org/WP99-03-HarperFatherAbsence.pdf. Accessed 6 July 2018.

Hartnet, C. S., Fingerman, K., & Birditt, K. S. (2016). *Without the ties that bind: Young adults who lack active parental relationships.* Ann Arbor: University of Michigan Population Studies Center Research Report. https://www.psc.isr.umich.edu/pubs/pdf/rr16-870.pdf. Accessed 6 July 2018.

Hewlett, S. A., & Luce, C. B. (2005). Off-ramps and on-ramps: Keeping talented women on the road to success. *Harvard Business Review*, March. https://hbr.org/2005/03/off-ramps-and-on-ramps-keeping-talented-women-on-the-road-to-success. Accessed 6 July 2018.

Hirshman, L. (2006). *Get to work: A manifesto for women of the world.* New York: Viking Books.

Hochschild, A. R. (2012). *The outsourced self: What happens when we pay others to live our lives for us.* New York: Henry Holt.

Kamminer, A. (2012, March 8). Jennifer Westfeldt and John Hamm give birth (to a movie). *The New York Times*, p. 128. http://www.nytimes.com/2012/03/11/magazine/jennifer-westfeldt-friends-with-kids.html. Accessed 6 July 2018.

Klein, T. P., Miranda, C., Nofi, E., & Bresgi, G. (2006). Parenting toddlers today: Ins and outs, ups and downs. Presentation at the Zero to Three Conference, Albuquerque.

Lang, K., & Zagorsky, J. (2001). Does growing up with an absent parent really hurt? *Journal of Human Resources, 36*(2), 253–273.

Lareau, A. (2002). Invisible inequality: Social class and childrearing in black families and white families. *American Sociological Review, 67*(5), 747–776. https://www.jstor.org/stable/3088916?seq=1#page_scan_tab_contents. Accessed 6 July 2018.

Last, J. V. (2014). *What to expect when no one's expecting.* New York: Encounter Books.

McLanahan, S., & Sandefur, G. (1997). *Growing up with a single parent.* Cambridge, MA: Harvard University Press.

Mead, R. (2006, April 26). The wives of others: Are stay-at-home mothers putting themselves – and feminism – at risk? *The New Yorker.* https://www.newyorker.com/magazine/2007/04/16/the-wives-of-others. Accessed 6 July 2018.

Mendle, J., et al. (2009). Associations between father absence and age of first sexual intercourse. *Child Development, 80*(5), 1463–1480. https://onlinelibrary.wiley.com/doi/abs/10.1111/j.1467-8624.2009.01345.x. Accessed 6 July 2018.

MSALT [Michigan Study of A&A Life Transition]. (2015). http://garp.education.uci.edu/msalt.html. Accessed 6 July 2018.

National Center for Fathering. (2009). One daughter's essay: Growing up without a Dad. https://www.youtube.com/watch?v=64V_NF43HPU. Accessed 6 July 2018.

Parker, K., & Stepler, R. (2017). As U.S. marriage rate hovers at 50%, education gap in marital status widens. Pew Research Center, September 14. http://www.pewresearch.org/fact-tank/2017/09/14/as-u-s-marriage-rate-hovers-at-50-education-gap-in-marital-status-widens/. Accessed 6 July 2018.

Pew Research Center. (2007). As marriage and parenthood drift apart, public is concerned about social impact. http://www.pewsocialtrends.org/2007/07/01/as-marriage-and-parenthood-drift-apart-public-is-concerned-about-social-impact/. Accessed 6 July 2018.

Plato. (n.d.). *The Republic*, Book V. https://tinyurl.com/yckx43a2. Accessed 6 July 2018.

Power to Decide, the campaign to prevent unplanned pregnancy (2018). National Statistics: New Jersey. https://powertodecide.org/what-we-do/information/national-state-data/national?state=newjersey. Accessed 6 July 2018.

Roosevelt, D. B. (2002). *Grandmère: A personal history of Eleanor Roosevelt*. Bolinas: Book Laboratory.

RWJF [Robert Wood Johnson Foundation]. (2018). National Survey of Families and Households, Wave 3: 2001–2003 (ICPSR 171). Health and Medical Care Archive, June 6, 2018. https://www.icpsr.umich.edu/icpsrweb/HMCA/studies/171. Accessed 6 July 2018.

Single Mothers by Choice. (n.d.). https://www.singlemothersbychoice.org/. Accessed 6 July 2018.

Slaughter, A.-M. (2012, July/August). Why women still can't have it all. *The Atlantic*. https://www.theatlantic.com/magazine/archive/2012/07/why-women-still-cant-have-it-all/309020/. Accessed 6 July 2018.

Terman, L. M. (1925). *Mental and physical traits of a thousand gifted children* (Genetic Studies of Genius) (Vol. 1). Stanford: Stanford University Press.

United States Census. (2018). America's families and living arrangements: 2017.

US Bureau of Labor Statistics. (2018, April 19). Employment characteristics of families – 2017. USDL-18-0589. https://www.bls.gov/news.release/pdf/famee.pdf. Accessed 6 July 2018. https://www.census.gov/data/tables/2017/demo/families/cps-2017.html. Accessed 6 July 2018.

Wilcox, W. B., & Wolfinger, N. H. (2017). Hey guys, put a ring on it. *National Review*, February 9, 2017. https://www.nationalreview.com/2017/02/marriage-benefits-men-financial-health-sex-divorce-caveat/. Accessed 6 July 2018.

Zero to Three. (2010, February 8). How to care for infants and toddlers in groups. https://www.zerotothree.org/resources/77-how-to-care-for-infants-and-toddlers-in-groups. Accessed 6 July 2018.

Chapter 10
The Rights and Needs of Newborn Babies and Young Children

> *There is no such thing as a baby ...*
> *A baby cannot exist alone but is essentially part*
> *of a relationship.*
> *The Child, the Family, and the Outside World*
>
> D. W. Winnicott, M.D. (1964)

Significant strides have been made to overcome blatant juvenile ageism even though it has not been formally acknowledged as a form of prejudice and discrimination. Childhood and adolescence are recognized as unique stages of development today. Still, the fact that a newborn baby is a unique human being — and a citizen — is not recognized in popular thought or most legal doctrines. This is not surprising. It took a long time for older children to gain recognition as human beings with basic rights.

Seeing a child as immature rather than as merely ignorant took shape in the eighteenth century. Rousseau and the Romantic poets dispelled the distorted view that children are miniature adults. The American Civil War established the civil rights of individual adults and created the opportunity for a vision of the civil rights of children and the role of the state in American life.

In 1870, the Illinois Supreme Court decision in People v. Turner extended due process protection to minors. It sets the stage throughout the United States for juvenile courts that were established in 1899 and expanded in the 1910s to administer payments to single mothers, a precursor of the federal Temporary Assistance to Needy Families program.

A wide-ranging "Save the Children" movement ushered in the twentieth century as the Century of the Child. The New York Society for the Prevention of Cruelty to Children had been formed in 1875. In 1909, the Swedish feminist Ellen Key (1909) published *The Century of the Child*. In her vision, babies would be conceived by loving parents. They would grow up in homes where mothers were ever present.

This vision dominated most of the first half of the 1900s. The aim was to map out a childhood in which children would acquire the "habit of happiness." This inspired the professional approach to childhood and adolescence through pediatrics, developmental psychology, child-centered education, child welfare, child and adolescent

© Springer Nature Switzerland AG 2019
J. C. Westman, *Dealing with Child Abuse and Neglect as Public Health Problems*, https://doi.org/10.1007/978-3-030-05897-5_10

psychology and psychiatry, and policy studies related to the young. Goldstein, Freud, and Solnit's classic book *Beyond the Best Interests of the Child* (Goldstein et al. 1979) set the tone for this era.

In the second half of the twentieth century, a sense arose that childhood was disappearing. The worlds of children and adults were merging again. Materially better off, children now often are expected to be independent and to adjust to a variety of family styles. Adolescents especially are wooed as major consumers. The more children act like adults in sports and in schools the better.

Underlying these developments is recognition of the rights of minors. These rights culminate in most adult legal rights being granted typically during late adolescence at the age of 18.

10.1   The Rights of Children

Rights have two distinct but related functions: to protect a person's freedoms and to fill important needs. The most important needs of children are protection from harm by others and themselves and to grow up to become productive citizens.

Minors lack the capacity and experience to marry, enter contracts, and bring lawsuits without adult approval and guidance. They are considered minors until they reach the age of majority at either 18 or 21, depending upon the state and the privileges. Until then, they are required to have legal and physical custodians, usually their parents. Since late adolescents are older than 18 and are regarded as legal adults in most ways, references to adolescent rights in this chapter are limited to early and middle adolescence.

When newborn babies and children were regarded as the property of their parents, they had no rights. Only their parents had rights based on the liberties and privacy of individuals. Now those parental rights are legal (acting on behalf of) and custodial (residential). Over the last century, minors have been accorded a series of moral and civil rights based on moral and civil rights that apply to all human beings.

10.2   Moral Rights of Minors

Moral rights reflect cultural values devoted to the common good and compassion for others. Immanuel Kant said that each human being "must always be treated as an end, not merely as a means." To treat another person as a means is to use that person to advance one's own interests. To treat another person as an end is to respect that person's dignity and autonomy. This distinction is especially important for young persons who are vulnerable to oppression and exploitation.

The traditional caretaker view of minor's moral rights was articulated in 1691 by the philosopher John Locke. According to him, all humans are "born infants, weak and helpless, without knowledge or understanding." Therefore, parents were "by the law of nature under an obligation to preserve, nourish, and educate the children they had begotten." In Locke's scheme, parents have the right to make choices for their children:

> Whilst [the child] is in an estate wherein he has no understanding of his own to direct his will, he is not to have any will of his own to follow.

Moral rights impose a duty to actively help a person. For example, a minor's moral right to education imposes a duty to provide that education.

Eglantyne Jebb, founder of the Save the Children Fund, began an effort to codify the moral rights of minors in 1922 in England's Charter of the Rights of the Child. The Charter spelled out the moral right of all minors to be protected from exploitation; to be given a chance for full physical, mental, and moral development; and to be taught to live a life of service. The League of Nations adopted the Charter in 1924 as the Geneva Declaration of the Rights of the Child.

In the United States, the moral rights of minors have been detailed in a variety of organizational creeds, children's bills of rights and White House Conferences on Children. Further declarations have come from the United Nations. These rights reflect reasonable expectations that minors will be given whatever they require to grow into healthy, functional adults. The United Nations Convention on the Rights of the Child adopted in 1989 states that all human beings are born with the following inherent civil rights (UN 1989):

- To survival
- To develop to the fullest
- To protection from harmful influences, abuse, and exploitation
- To participate fully in family, cultural, and social life

Whenever policymakers express their hopes for children, they effectively conclude that children have a moral right to competent parents and specifically to not live in protracted foster care or institutions. When parents and other persons make decisions for a child, they act as fiduciary custodians. They are expected to put themselves in the child's position and place the child's interests above their own. The contemporary challenge is to apply the same principles to newborn babies.

10.3   The Civil Rights of Minors

Moral rights are not enough to protect minors from abuse and neglect. For this reason, certain moral rights of minors have become legal civil rights. Civil rights spring from the seventeenth and eighteenth centuries' reformist theories of human rights, the same ideals that inspired the English, American, and French Revolutions. They guarantee all citizens equal protection under the law regardless of race, religion, gender, age, or disability, equal exercise of the privileges of citizenship, and equal participation in community life. Newborn babies are equal in the sense that they are entitled to as much respect for their rights as are adults.

Moral rights became enforceable civil rights for minorities and women only through great effort and vigilance. Even more effort and vigilance is required to enforce important civil rights for minors, especially for newborn babies. For the first time in history, we are poised to specify rights for minors in positive terms. Of course, these civil rights are based on their developmental needs and capacities rather than their wishes.

Adult civil rights that apply to minors include freedom from racial and gender discrimination, the right to life and personal security, freedom from slavery and involuntary servitude, and freedom from cruel, inhuman, or degrading treatment and punishment. In 2005, the US Supreme Court recognized the relative incapacity of minors and ruled that the execution of minors violates the cruel and unusual punishment clause of the Eighth Amendment.

The gradual emergence of minors' civil rights in the United States began through different treatment in criminal matters. The first juvenile court was established in 1899 in Cook County, Illinois. Because existing courts were not adequately rehabilitating juveniles, the US Supreme Court ruling in 1967 in In re Gault mandated due process to provide Constitutional protections for them. Unfortunately, this did not actually improve the courts' abilities to help juveniles as much as intended.

Minors' civil rights progressed from child labor, child neglect and abuse, and education laws to the idea that children have the right to environments that offer reasonable opportunities for healthy development. These include adequate nutrition, housing, recreation, and health care as well as love, security, education, and protection from abuse and discrimination.

These rights do not include certain adult rights such as the right to privacy, the right to confidentiality, and the right to make their own choices on vital matters. All of this boils down to the right to have competent parents. Competent parenting actually is an enforceable affirmative civil right because incompetent parenting is a cause for state intervention through child abuse and neglect laws. These laws allow for the termination of parental rights by the state.

In 1968, in Ginsberg v. New York, the US Supreme Court recognized society's interest in protecting minors from circumstances that might prevent them from becoming responsible citizens:

> The state also has an independent interest in the wellbeing of its youth...to protect the welfare of children ... safeguarded from abuses which might prevent their growth into free and independent well-developed ... citizens.

Stated positively, minors have a civil right to nurturance, to protection, and to make certain choices through age-grading statutes. Still, the fact that parental rights are based on the right of minors to have competent parents is not yet fully appreciated by courts or the public.

The civil right of minors to competent parents is more important than adult rights to freedom of actions because of the adverse consequences incompetent parents impose on our society. Adults' rights benefit individuals and are the backbone of our democratic society, but minors' rights are essential for our society's survival and prosperity. Our society's well-being depends on protecting and nurturing our young so that they can become responsible citizens.

10.4   The Right to Competent Parents

None of us have a moral right to succeed. In fact, we have a right to fail unless our failure adversely affects other people. The failures of parents do affect others, including their children and society, and fly in the face of children's rights to competent parents. A person's freedom to fail therefore faces an exception when that person is a parent.

The legal right of newborn babies to competent parents stems from the fact that incompetent parents justify state intervention and possible termination of parental rights. Because our society is paying an ever larger share of the cost of rearing, educating, and treating neglected and abused children, we all have a financial stake in competent parents.

Public decisionmaking needs to acknowledge the interests of children and that parents usually protect those interests best. But when a parent's inability to do so is evident before childbirth, the state is obligated by existing child abuse and neglect statutes to intervene preemptively.

Our society must value newborn babies enough to protect their rights to competent parents and to enforce its expectations of parenthood before childbirth. Whether or not a pregnancy was planned, a person's decision to enter parenthood should be based on a newborn's right to a competent parent before the child is born. Action should not be delayed until after childbirth when maternal and paternal instincts, hormones, and ideologically and fantasy-based emotions impede problem solving and decisionmaking.

10.5   The Developmental Needs of Babies

The notion that all babies require is feeding and diapering prevails in popular thought and public policies. This is reflected in the use of the term caregiving rather than parenting as the primary need of babies and toddlers. The fact that they are interacting, learning human beings seeking to form relationships with their parents from the day of birth has not taken solid root.

Babies usually are seen as objects to be adored and cared for. This view allows us to overlook the fact that a difficult birth and time in intensive care, and even circumcision, are traumatic for newborns. It makes it possible to ignore the baby while dealing with the crisis of adolescent childbirth, including establishing paternity. It makes it possible to presume that baby boys aren't affected by the pain of circumcision. It makes it possible to ignore the connection between baby-parent love and loving adult relationships in later life. It makes it possible to successfully market videos for babies that absorb their attention and ensnare them with "infotainment" rather than exploring their world on their own.

The fact that their development as human beings depends on enduring parent attachments formed through parent-child interactions is not fully appreciated by the general public in part because parenthood cannot compete with less demanding and more materially rewarding activities. Actually, newborn babies are interacting persons in every sense of the word. They analyze and respond to sounds. They stop feeding to listen to something. When they hear other babies cry, they usually cry with them. They might stop crying on hearing a recording of their own voice. They gaze deeply into their mothers' eyes. They closely watch their mothers. They are upset when their mothers wear expressionless masks or when their mothers are depressed. They hunger for interaction with humans who are motivated to bond with them and can fill their survival needs. Without a doubt, they are human beings … they are persons.

10.6   Attachment Bonding

Historians, archeologists, and anthropologists building on the work of Charles Darwin have described the human capacity for attachment bonding, cooperation, and altruism from early life. Animal research suggests that bonding between mother and baby is encoded through genes in addition to the usual memory process. The bonding process tempers self-assertive-individual-survival instincts with integrative-species-survival instincts.

While competition is a key motivator in human affairs, cooperation is even more important. The viability of interpersonal relationships and market economies depend upon our virtuous natures. Higher brain centers evolved to ensure species survival through attachment bonding between parents and children and among intimate groups. These trust-inducing advantages contributed to neurological attachment bonding systems fostered by hormones.

The attachment bonding process begins before birth. Research on lifetime health records reveals that characteristics in later life are affected by our experiences in the womb. A classic example was the retarded growth of women who were low-birth-weight newborns during the Dutch Hunger Winter of 1944–1945 and who later gave birth to smaller babies themselves even with adequate nutrition during their pregnancies (Stein et al. 1975).

Newborn babies seek attachment bonds. They can form close relationships, express themselves forcefully, show preferences, form memories, and influence people from day 1. They show their thoughts when they reach out, give an inquisitive look, frown, scream in protest, gurgle in satisfaction, or gasp in excitement. They listen intently to their mothers' voices, which they readily distinguish from other voices. They engage in complex activities that integrate their senses and enable learning.

The psychologist John Bowlby's groundbreaking theory of attachment bonding borrows from cybernetics, the study of how mechanical and biological systems self-regulate to achieve goals as their external and internal environments change (Bretherton 1992). Attachment theory begins with the idea that two basic goals guide young children's behavior: safety and exploration. A child who stays safe survives; a child who explores develops the intelligence and skills needed for adult life.

These needs often oppose each other, so they are regulated by a cybernetic thermostat that monitors safety. When safe, a child explores and plays. When safety is uncertain, a switch is thrown that triggers fear and withdrawal. The attachment bonding process allows children to handle these emotions by internalizing models of their caregivers. As they mature, these working models become their self-regulating thermostats. Four kinds of interactions develop the working models children and parents build of each other.

- First is the succoring bonding system present at birth. It extends from infancy into adolescence and seeks bonding with parents.
- Second is the affiliative bonding system, which emerges during early childhood attachment bonding and continues into adulthood to sustain friendships.
- Third is the sexual bonding system, which becomes prominent after puberty, continues through adult life, and fosters romantic relationships.
- Fourth is the nurturing bonding system, which flowers after puberty, continues throughout life, and fosters bonding to a child and intimate relationships between adults.

Development of the nurturing bonding system builds on the succoring and affiliative systems. In turn, those systems depend on having been nurtured in the intertwining parent-child relationship. The capacities for each system are present during early life and emerge more fully at successive levels of development. Each system is based on human needs that persist throughout life.

These systems ensure that individuals survive and produce progeny. Many people lead full lives without reproducing, but the evolutionary purpose of their interpersonal bonding is reproduction, not just companionship or sexual gratification. Stable family relationships depend upon dampening the self-assertive individual-survival instincts expressed through the succoring and sexual bonding systems. This is achieved by the integrative-species-survival instincts of the affiliative and nurturant bonding systems.

10.6.1   Succoring Bonding System

A baby's succoring bonding system seeks essential caregiving for the baby's physical survival through such activities as feeding and cuddling. As seen in orphanages, without attachment bonding babies fail to thrive physically and even die. Templates for succoring bonding to mother and father images appear to be genetically programmed. Interactions with additional caregivers can help babies gauge the intentions of others and elicit their care, which also can be important for survival.

Mothers who give birth are deeply attached to the human beings who were in their bodies. Prenatal exposure to the mother's voice and odors primes a newborn to respond preferentially to a birth mother. Human babies recognize the sight, sounds, smell, and touch of their mothers but apparently do not recognize their fathers the same way.

At first attachment bonding is unidirectional. Over time working models of the parent are built into the baby's brain just as images of the baby are encoded in the parent's brain. A baby's distress triggers caregiving instincts in the parent. A baby's drive for succorance is reinforced by receiving nurturing from the person to whom the baby attaches.

Nurturing instincts insure that mothers are devoted to their newborns. After birth, the baby is the center of a breast-feeding mother's life. Physical transformations in her body continue after birth. Nurturing her baby produces hormones and inscribes new pathways in her brain that lower the amount of stimulation needed to elicit maternal responses. Breastfeeding releases oxytocin with a relaxing effect. Within days a mother can pick out her own baby's clothes by smell alone.

Without DNA testing, fathers have no way of being certain about their parentage other than what they believe to be true. Still, a strongly attached father can be more important to his baby's well-being than a weakly attached mother.

10.6.2   Affiliative Bonding System

The affiliative bonding system favors the cooperative behavior essential for the survival of the species. Also referred to as reciprocal bonding, affiliative bonding builds on one-way succoring bonding in babies and nurturant bonding in their parents. It goes beyond a child's instinctive quest for security and a parent's instincts to nurture and protect. It involves a range of two-way dimensions that include intimacy, shared humor, and positive emotions.

A child succoringly attaches to a caregiver and affiliatively bonds through shared interactions with a caregiver. A parent nurturingly bonds with a child by responding to the child's succoring attachment. A child's initial succoring attachment grows into affiliative bonding. However, babies do not become succoringly or affiliatively bonded with genetic mothers and fathers who do not interact intimately with them.

Babies and children form succoring and affiliative bonds with adoptive parents who nurture them. Children who discover they have been adopted have socially conditioned reactions, but they do not automatically shift their bonding relationships from their adoptive parents to their genetic ones. Life experience rather than genes creates succoring and affiliative parent-child bonding.

A deep emotional bond with genetic relatives also is not based on genes. It comes from reciprocal affiliative bonding that takes place through child-parent and sibling relationships. Affiliative attachment bonds are imprinted in the brain. Adoptive parents are the real parents through their succoring attachment and affiliative bonds with their children.

Affiliatively bonded adults and children build evolving images in each other's brains. They sense and respond to each other's needs. Reciprocal interactions with caregivers develop a child's capacity for higher mental functions, empathy, compassion, and resilience … in essence, they develop the child's mind.

10.6.3 Sexual Bonding System

The sexual bonding system appears early in life in the form of the Electra and Oedipal complexes. These complexes motivate attachment bonding with the parent of the opposite sex and rivalry with the parent of the same sex. Sexual feelings and fantasies later evolve during adolescence with the eventual goal of mating and reproduction.

Lustful craving is the basic motivation for sexual union. Lust does not automatically result in romantic passion nor the urge to attach to a mating partner. Lust's capriciousness might be part of nature's plan. It enabled our ancestors to follow two complementary reproductive strategies. If a male had one mate and two children by a female from a different band, he would double his descendants. Likewise, a female who had a mate and became involved with another male might bear the latter's baby and acquire extra food and protection for her children.

Romantic passion, the elation and obsession associated with being in love, focuses courtship on one individual at a time. The process focuses the evolutionary precious time and energy spent on mating and reproduction.

Passionate love's symptoms overlap with those of heroin (euphoric well-being) and cocaine (energetic euphoria). When passion is spurned or thwarted, the brain reacts with negative feelings like despair, depression, and rage, all of which are similar to withdrawal symptoms from heroin or cocaine usage. Most commonly, the need for passionate love eventually diminishes as affiliative bonding strengthens attachment bonding between a couple.

10.6.4 Nurturing Bonding System

The nurturing bonding system first appears in young children's caregiving impulses. When fully expressed in parenthood and adult companionship, it fulfills the reproductive cycle.

Romantic passion based on testosterone and estrogens does not necessarily turn into nurturant attachment. They are separate processes and follow different patterns. Under the influence of oxytocin, nurturing attachment grows slowly over time as lovers rely upon, care for, and deepen the trust between them. Passionate love is like fire. Nurturing love is like a growing vine that intertwines two people. Parent-child and enduring intimate adult relationships are both examples of this kind of love. Nurturing attachment between them motivates partners to stay together long enough to rear their young. When disrupted, it can cause pain. The desire for nurturing attachment generally is stronger in females than in males.

Homo sapiens is a social species full of emotions finely tuned for loving, helping, sharing, and intertwining our lives. There are as many ways to have enduring companionship attachments as there are couples. Underlying them all is the willingness to compromise with and tolerate a partner as well as to nurture each other.

10.6.5   Attachment Styles

Attachment styles emerge gradually over time. A child with a particular temperament makes bids for nurturance. A mother with a particular temperament responds or does not respond based on her mood, how overworked she is, or which childrearing expert she has been reading. Children with sunny dispositions and upbeat mothers are likely to develop secure attachment bonds. Still, a dedicated mother can overcome her own and/or her child's less pleasant disposition and foster secure attachment bonding.

A parent's capacity to respond to the emotional and mental states of a newborn baby is the foundation of secure attachment bonding. These mutual experiences develop a baby's reflective capacity and create an internal sense of cohesion and interpersonal connection. Over time, babies and young children build what John Bowlby called internal working models of themselves, their parents, and their relationships with others. This self-organizing internal model of a mother provides a sense of security when the mother is not present.

Children of parents who are empathic, set firm limits, and emphasize the rights and welfare of others show high levels of pro-social and compassionate behaviors. Genetic differences also play a role. In contrast, in dysfunctional families children can become frightened or angry. They can lash out or turn away from others. In steeling themselves against their own emotional pain, they become inured to the pain of others.

10.7   The Developing Mind

We do not ordinarily think of ourselves this way, but each one of us is a complicated self-organizing system with self-organizing subsystems including the central nervous system...the seat of the mind. The development of a child's brain depends upon communication between the minds of parent and child. It occurs through observation and interaction with more knowledgeable members of the culture throughout childhood. These connections involve an energetic resonance in which information flows freely. This learning process can be exhilarating for both child and adult.

Stable mental images are formed in babies' brains as they interact with their caregivers. A baby and mother recognize each other's faces and smile, giving the baby a secure feeling. Babies form images of their parents' bodies, personalities, and behavior as their minds are shaped by their parents.

A child learns to regulate emotional states in response to parental constraints. The orbitofrontal cortex in the brain operates like a clutch that disengages the sympathetic nervous system (the accelerator) and activates the parasympathetic system (the brakes). This part of the brain is especially sensitive to face-to-face communication. This is why eye-to-eye contact between parent and child helps set effective limits. The meaning of the word "no" is conveyed more clearly with eye contact than by shouting across a room. This is the basis for the parenting limit-setting maxim: "Use your feet instead of your mouth."

Learning that wishes are not automatically gratified and that one's mind and a parent's mind are separate helps a child learn self-control as well as modulate emotions and behavior in pro-social ways. The clash of separate minds and wills is essential to mental and social development.

10.7.1   Self-Generated Play

Self-generated, creative play enriches personal growth and the capacity for enjoyment and creativity later. The world of symbolic meaning creates awareness that one has a subjective experience…a mind of one's own. Creative imagination-stimulating pretending crystallizes a child's ideas so that the ideas become thoughts that can be thought about. When children grasp the fact that minds are independent, they acquire their own minds. They expand their own creative imaginations.

Then the insight dawns that the child is one among others. From this time on, a child can think about other people as individuals who have their own experiences. At this point, children enter society and culture. Young children who passively view television may well be less imaginative and empathic than those who engage in self-generated, creative play.

10.7.2   Us/Them Memes

The feelings associated with relationships that are not based on attachment bonding are based on the genetic capacity to form us/them feelings. These feelings are culturally transmitted through behavioral and feeling patterns called memes, which are ingrained mental images of our relationships that become a part of our brain structures.

Perceptions of genetic relatives are based more on our experiences with them through memes than on genes. The biological mechanisms of memes permit us to have perceptions of genetic ties even though there is no actual genetic connection. Our tribal forbearers relied heavily on the perception of genetic ties even when there were none. As time went on, the disadvantages of mating with close genetic relatives became evident and created the need to identify actual genetic kin and avoid mating with them.

An example of how kinship feelings can crop up is when a person learns of a genetic connection to another person and experiences a visceral feeling. This is an us/them feeling and is not the same as feelings associated with attachment bonding. Instead it is based on memes.

Us/them meme feelings can shift away from individuals as our perceptions of them change. For example, friendships shift depending on how attitudes between people evolve. Marriages endure because nurturant bonds develop between couples, not just because of romantic or affiliative feelings or us/them meme codes.

The emotions involved in genetic and adoptive kinship are based on secure attachment bonding rather than on genes or on us/them memes. As adopted children and their parents know, mutual love is based on attachment bonding to each other and has nothing to do with genes.

10.7.3 *Special Considerations in Father Relationships*

Most children enjoy affiliative and, to a lesser degree than with their mothers, succoring attachment bonding with fathers. Some receive inconsistent support, while others are adversely affected by their father's behavior. Still others lose their fathers early in life. Some children have high levels of involvement with males other than their genetic fathers, like grandfathers and uncles.

Fathers can provide emotional support to mothers and participate in childcare whether they live with the mother or not. Fathers also can link children to their extended families and community resources. Fathers are more likely to engage children in physical and stimulating play while mothers tend to spend more time in verbal activities.

10.8 Honoring Children's Rights

Children have come a long way from when they were seen as miniature adults and adolescence was not recognized as a developmental stage in life. We are evolving from a baseline of extreme prejudice and discrimination against children…especially against newborns, who still can be murdered at parents' discretion in some parts of the world. When children were regarded as property, they had no rights at all. Now they have moral and civil rights. Our society has taken decisive steps toward overcoming juvenile ageism.

At the same time, the notion that babies need only feeding and diapering still prevails in popular thought and public policies. The facts that babies are interacting, learning human beings and that their development depends on enduring parental attachments are not fully appreciated.

The development of the brain depends upon communication between the minds of parent and child. Babies internalize working models of their parents; in this way, their developing minds are shaped by their parents' more mature minds and actions.

Children's rights spring from human rights that specify the minimum standards of civilized behavior. They all hinge on the right to competent parents. Competent parenthood rests upon attachment bonds that promote self-respect, self-confidence and resiliency in both children and their parents. Although parental rights come from the Constitutional protection of the privacy of the family and individual liberty, they really reflect legal and physical custodial duties essential for the survival of our species and our nation. Parental rights deserve careful consideration.

References

Bretherton, I. (1992). The origins of attachment theory: John Bowlby and Mary Ainsworth. *Developmental Psychology, 28*, 759–775.

Goldstein, J., Freud, A., & Solnit, A. J. (1979). *Beyond the best interests of the child*. New York: The Free Press.

Key, E. (1909). *The century of the child*. New York: G. P. Putnam & Sons.

Stein, Z., Susser, M., Saenger, G., & Marolla, F. (1975). *Famine and human development: The Dutch hunger winter of 1944–1945*. New York: Oxford University Press.

United Nations. (1989). Convention on the rights of the child, New York. https://treaties.un.org/pages/ViewDetails.aspx?src=IND&mtdsg_no=IV-11&chapter=4&lang=en. Accessed 6 July 2018.

Winnicott, D. W. (1964). *The child, the family, and the outside world*. New York: Pelican.

Chapter 11
The Rights of Parents

> *Today we may not blame parents for being largely instrumental in getting their boys and girls into trouble. But twenty or thirty years from now, we will have to point our finger against those parents who, because of neglect or ignorance, wittingly or unwittingly bring out the worst in their children.*
>
> David Abrahamson, Who Are the Guilty? (1952)

The idea that individuals have rights springs from the vulnerability of every human being in the face of stronger forces. Our *Declaration of Independence* and *Constitution* are based on the idea that the purpose of government is not to protect the elite, nor to facilitate greed or self-interest nor to promote a religious group's agenda. Its purpose is to guarantee certain inalienable human rights for all people including our nation's posterity … our young citizens.

Most of us presume that parents have rights that give them exclusive power over their children, especially newborn babies. But the need to specify those rights only arises when things go wrong in families and in child-serving institutions. Unfortunately, the emotionally charged issue of parental rights arises quite often today. Parents compel state intervention when they neglect and/or abuse or dispute custody of their children. Minors give birth. Too many child-serving institutions are overburdened and unable to function effectively.

Even defining who is a parent can be complicated. With surrogate birth and artificial insemination, defining a mother and a father can be complicated. By eliminating the ambiguous term "natural parent" from its rules for establishing a legal parent-child relationship, the Uniform Parentage Act encourages courts to focus on the precise relationship a female or male has to a child. Is the relationship of each mother and father (1) genetic, (2) birth (mother only), (3) functional, (4) stepparent, or (5) adoptive? A single child could have as many as nine different persons legally recognized as a parent by adding (6) foster, (7) step, (8) surrogate, and (9) sperm or egg donor (Parentage Act 2017).

© Springer Nature Switzerland AG 2019
J. C. Westman, *Dealing with Child Abuse and Neglect as Public Health Problems*, https://doi.org/10.1007/978-3-030-05897-5_11

11.1   Parental Rights

Because of their obligations to their children, parents need rights or prerogatives to protect and fulfill the human rights of their children. Unfortunately, contemporary talk about human rights usually emphasizes the rights to benefits and overlooks the responsibilities that accompany those rights.

In the past, children have been treated as the personal property of their parents. Under Roman law, the *patria potestas* doctrine gave fathers life and death power over their children. To this day, the popular presumption is that children belong to their parents.

In contrast, since The Enlightenment of the eighteenth century, parenthood in Western cultures has been seen as a contract between parents and society by philosophers and evolving legal codes. Parents are awarded rights in exchange for discharging their responsibilities.

John Locke in the seventeenth century and William Blackstone in the eighteenth century held that parental rights and powers arise from their duty to care for their offspring. They recognized that no society can survive unless its children grow up to be responsible, productive citizens. Children also have the right to be raised without unjustified interference by the state. Taken together, these rights are called the right of family integrity. Both Locke and Blackstone held that, if a choice is forced upon society, it is more important to protect the rights of children than to protect the rights of adults.

Every man and every woman has a natural and Constitutional right to procreate. This principle could be reasonably applied when the onset of menarche was between 16 and 18. Now that menarche appears on average at the age of 12, we must ask if every girl and boy has a natural and Constitutional right to procreate. In the light of this question, the need for careful thought about parental rights and responsibilities is intensified.

11.2   The Child-Parent Relationship

James Garbarino (1995), professor of psychology at Loyola University Chicago, points out that parental rights are influenced by personal and public views of child-parent relationships. Are children:

- The private property of parents
- Members of families with no direct link to the state
- Citizens with a primary relationship with the state

11.2.1   Children as Private Property

Parental rights have become the most protected and cherished of all Constitutional rights. They are based on the natural right to beget children and the likelihood that affection leads parents to act in the best interests of their children. The Fourth Amendment's protection of the privacy of the home and the Fourteenth Amendment's due process clause are interpreted to give parents legal and physical custody of their children. The popular presumption that children are the property of their parents therefore is understandable.

In the 1995 Congress, a Parental Rights and Responsibilities Act was introduced. It would have created a Constitutional amendment specifying absolute parental rights. It did not gather support because the legal system already respects parental rights. It also would have made protecting children from neglect and abuse more difficult.

In spite of strongly held beliefs to the contrary, the legal system no longer considers children as property. There even is a genetic basis for the legal position that parents do not own their children. The genes we give them are not our own. Our own genes were mixed when they were transmitted to us by our parents. Our genes are beyond our control. We really do not own them. They extend back through previous generations and potentially forward into future generations. We are only the temporary custodians of our own genes and of our children.

Mary Lyndon Shanley (2001), professor of political science at Vassar College, holds that an individual's right to reproduce and a parent's wishes cannot be the primary foundation of family law (Shanley 2001). The primary focus must be on children's needs and interests. The parent-child relationship is one of stewardship. Parental authority involves responsibilities beyond the parent's own wishes.

Moreover, our legal system is based on the principle that no individual is entitled to own another human being. Guardians of incompetent adults are agents, not owners, of those persons. In the same way, the childrearing rights of parents consist of (1) the guardianship right (legal custody) to make decisions on behalf of a child and (2) the right to physical custody of the child. These rights are based on a child's interests and needs rather than ownership of the child. We certainly do not own our children.

11.2.2   Children as Family Members

Children are generally regarded as family members with no direct link to the state. The concept of parental rights sprang from traditions and Constitutional precedents that endow genetic and adoptive parents with special rights.

Parental rights are legal prerogatives based on the moral and civil rights of children to be nurtured and protected. They are based on the assumption that parents can best decide how to raise a child without undue interference by the state. Without a voluntary or involuntary forfeiture of parental duties, the state cannot permanently remove children from their parents' custody to seek a better home for them unless there has been a legal termination of parental rights.

11.2.3   Children as Citizens

Two trends have added the view of a child as a citizen. The first is the growing emphasis on the right of children to grow up without neglect or abuse. The second is increased limitations on parental control seen in child neglect and abuse laws, child labor laws, mandatory education laws, adolescent healthcare policies, and parental responsibility laws. When parents do not fulfill their responsibilities, child protection services intervene, and governmental agencies can assume legal and physical custody. Then the child's primary relationship is with the state as custodian.

Like other guardians, parents have the legal prerogative to make stewardship decisions. Society generally defers to their authority. The challenge is to encourage parents to act in the interests of their children rather than in their own selfish interests. Toward this end, lawmakers rely on persuasion and education to help parents fulfill their obligations. Because they are unresponsive to persuasion and education, some parents require legal interventions before and after a baby is born.

11.3   Parent-Society Contract

James Dwyer (2009), professor of law at William and Mary University, affirms that parental rights do not have a direct Constitutional basis. The emergence of children's rights reflects this position; our society has progressively and empirically limited the control parents have over their children's lives.

Dwyer endorses the Enlightenment view that persons who conceive and give birth enter an implicit contract with society to raise their children as responsible citizens. Damage caused by maltreatment extends beyond the individuals involved and gives our society a compelling interest in the wellbeing of our young.

Mark Vopat (2015), professor of philosophy at Youngstown State University, also holds that a parent's obligations derive from an implicit contract with the state beyond the child. This Parent-Society Contract provides a strong moral imperative for public efforts that ensure every child's safety and quality of life. Since a contract implies mutual obligations, the parents and society are accountable to each other. The government's role is reflected in debates about:

- Child wellbeing. Is it an entitlement? A privilege? A tool for social control? The trend is to view it as an entitlement.

- Adolescent childbirth. Who has legal and physical custody of a minor's newborn baby? Strictly speaking no one, but relatives and government policies support minor parents by default.
- Financial support. Is financial responsibility for a child purely a private matter or a public responsibility? Both. Federal and state laws mandate childrearing benefits in addition to financial child support from parents and sometimes grandparents, as in Wisconsin.

In the Parent-Society Contract, government plays a vital role in supporting parents in rearing children and preventing maltreatment. The intimacy involved in family relationships cannot be provided by the state. It is the duty of families to rear children. Still, state and local governments are responsible for providing schools and safe neighborhoods to support childrearing. They can provide health insurance, tax deductions and welfare benefits as well.

Parents really do not need specifically defined rights. They have prerogatives that flow from their children's rights. Unfortunately, parental prerogatives and children's rights do not fit well in contemporary society. As examples, workplaces offer little accommodation for parents' childrearing duties, and, when children are held indefinitely in supposedly temporary foster care, their right to competent parents is unfulfilled.

Public policies must recognize that children have the right to be cared for by persons with an enduring commitment to, and the capacity for, parenthood. Public policies also need to recognize that in the Parent-Society Contract, society must ensure that parents have access to essential childrearing resources. The parental rights debate would be resolved by shifting it from children as property to parenthood as a career. Parenthood is a Parent-Society Contract-based career with prerogatives derived from the responsibility to nurture a child and to advocate for the child's interests.

Being the loving mother or father of a child does not necessarily mean that one is qualified for legal and physical custodial rights. Parental love is insufficient for healthy child development. A minor or developmentally disabled person can be a loving mother or father without having parental rights. Persons even remain a mother or a father of a child after parental rights have been terminated and other parents have assumed motherhood and fatherhood roles through adoption or kinship care.

11.3.1 The Rights of Mothers

The laws of every state give the woman or girl who conceives and bears a child automatic recognition as the legal mother. Giving birth follows the physical relationship formed during pregnancy. These state laws reflect an appropriately strong bias in favor of birth mothers, especially those who care for and form attachment bonds with their babies. This is complicated by surrogates who are not genetic mothers but who have a prenatal physical relationship with a newborn.

States seldom challenge genetic/birth motherhood unless compelling circumstances arise, such as a Child in Need of Protective Services petition filed before childbirth. Even in such cases, a newborn baby may be placed in foster care under state custody with the intention of rehabilitating the genetic/birth mother. This intent usually is not realized. A similar situation exists with children whose mothers are incarcerated with the expectation of maintaining the mothers' custody of their children. A 2009 study by Volunteers of America Through the Eyes of a Child: Life with a Mother in Prison revealed that after release of their mothers from prison, 81% of their children remained with their caregivers and did not live with their mothers (Volunteers of America 2018).

Women and girls who give birth can decline parenthood by voluntary revocation of their parental rights through a Termination of Parental Rights proceeding to allow for adoption. Paradoxically, implicit recognition that minors do not have the judgment required for parenthood is reflected in the fact that minors require a guardian ad litem in order to terminate their parental rights and an adult or institutional payee to receive Temporary Aid to Families with Dependent Children (TANF) benefits. An involuntary Termination of Parental Rights can be initiated after reasonable efforts to help parents meet return conditions have failed. Mothers' parental rights also can be terminated automatically at childbirth under circumstances such as previous involuntary terminations or murder of a sibling. In some states, third parties like foster parents can petition for the termination of genetic parental rights.

11.3.2   The Rights of Fathers

Unlike maternity, substantial Constitutional guidance has been provided for states in determining paternity. States must insure that men have the opportunity to seek to establish paternity. A genetic connection and a relationship with a child (or the effort to establish one) are necessary for Constitutional protection of a paternity claim.

To claim parental rights, males must register with putative father registries within varying time frames. Agencies are required to notify putative fathers of the mothers' adoption plans. Questions arise about the feasibility of making fathers aware of their need to register. In situations where genetic fathers do not want to acknowledge fatherhood, state agencies try to establish paternity through genetic testing, other biological evidence, or acknowledgment by the mother or the father in order to seek child support payments.

A father's genetic tie can be overridden when a child's interests are better served by a man who is married to the mother and who has established a relationship with the child. In the 1989 US Supreme Court case Michael H. v. Gerald D., the genetic father of a child produced during an adulterous relationship was denied paternity in favor of the father who actually was raising the child.

11.3.3 Parental Liability

The common-law doctrine of parental immunity has maintained that, in the absence of willful and wanton misconduct, children cannot sue their parents for negligence. In response to the magnitude of child neglect and abuse, most states and courts are beginning to define parental liability. As long ago as 1963, an Illinois Appeals Court heard Zepeda v. Zepeda in which a child sued his father for having caused him to be born out of wedlock. Although that suit was unsuccessful, it raised the issue of a child's legal right to be wanted, loved, and nurtured...in essence, to be competently parented.

Children have successfully sued their parents for negligence and have brought actions against third parties who alienate a parent from the family. In 1992 in Orlando, Florida, 11-year-old Gregory Kingsley legally "divorced" his mother so he could be adopted by his foster parents (Jill et al. 2012).

11.3.4 The Parens Patriae Doctrine

The most significant fact justifying state involvement is that children do not choose the families into which they are born. The *parens patriae* doctrine justifies state intervention as a part of the Parent-Society Contract. *Parens patriae* is Latin for "father of the people." The doctrine grants the inherent power and authority of the state to protect people who are legally unable to act on their own behalf. It gives state courts the ultimate power to terminate parental rights and is based on three assumptions:

- Childhood and adolescence are periods of dependency and require supervision.
- The family is of primary importance, but the state should play a role in a child's education and intervene when the family fails to provide adequate nurturance, moral training, or supervision.
- When parents disagree or fail to exercise their authority, the appropriate authority to determine a child's or an adolescent's interests is a public official.

The *parens patriae* doctrine empowers the state to compel parents and minors to act in ways that are beneficial to society. It never presumed that the state would assume parenting functions. Instead, the state is responsible for protecting the "best interests" of children under the guidance of two principles:

- The wellbeing of society depends upon children being educated and not being exploited.
- A child's developmental needs for nurturance and protection are defined by child neglect and abuse statutes.

A 1985 decision by Canada's Supreme Court made a child's welfare paramount in disputes between genetic parents and third parties. In King v. Low, the Court stated that although the genetic parents' claims would receive serious consideration, they must give way to the best interests of the children when the children have developed close psychological ties with another individual. This view is taking hold in American courts as well.

Our legal system distinguishes between what parents can do to themselves and what they can do to their children. For example, parents can refuse essential medical treatment themselves but usually are not allowed to do the same with their children. They also are not permitted to physically harm their children, nor can they allow children to physically harm themselves.

Parents who fail to provide a minimum level of care, who abandon their children, or who fail to provide supervision can be found guilty of neglect. Parents who physically, emotionally, or sexually abuse their children can be found guilty of abuse. Parents who have been convicted of a serious crime, who abuse drugs or alcohol, or who cannot meet return conditions after their children have been removed can be found unfit as parents. When persons cannot be persuaded or educated to become competent parents within a certain period of time, parental rights can be terminated to enable adoption.

11.3.5   State Liability

Despite the *parens patriae* doctrine, the liability of the state if it does not protect minors has not been clearly defined. In 1989, the US Supreme Court ruled in DeShaney v. Winnebago County Department of Social Services that the state is not required by the Fourteenth Amendment to protect the life, liberty, or property of its citizens against invasion by private actors (Smith v. Alameda County Social Services Agency 1979).

Joshua DeShaney suffered brain damage from repeated beatings by his father at the age of 4. As a result, Joshua was expected to remain institutionalized for life. The US Supreme Court rejected arguments that the state had a duty to protect Joshua because it once placed him in foster care and later because social workers suspected he was being abused by his father but took no action. It held that only "when the state takes a person into its custody and holds him there against his will" does the Fourteenth Amendment due process clause require officials to take responsibility for the individual's safety and wellbeing. At the same time, the Court did not rule out the possibility that the state acquired a duty to protect Joshua under tort law.

An appellate court in California upheld a local court's dismissal of a suit by a 17-year-old who alleged damage by mismanagement of his adoption as a newborn (Smith v. Alameda County Social Services Agency 1979). At the age of 17, Dennis Smith filed a complaint against the Alameda County Social Services Department alleging the agency was liable for damages because it failed to find an adoptive home when his mother gave him to the Department for the purpose of adoption shortly after his birth. The Department placed Dennis in a series of foster homes, but no one adopted him.

Dennis claimed that the Department negligently or intentionally failed to take reasonable actions to bring about his adoption. Therefore, he was deprived of proper and effective parental care and guidance and a secure family environment. Dennis alleged that this caused him mental and emotional damage.

The dismissal of Dennis' complaint was upheld in appellate court on a number of grounds, including the difficulty in directly linking his damage to the failure to arrange for his adoption. The court implied that liability could result with more convincing links between early life experience and later outcomes.

Cook County, Illinois, settled a claim out of court by an 18-year-old boy over the negligence of county social workers. In this case, the link between professional practices and damage to Billy Nichols apparently was made effectively (Gorner 1981; Westman 2007). In December of 1981, attorneys for the State of Illinois and Cook County paid $150,000 in an out-of-court settlement of a suit of a former dependent child, Billy Nichols, who had been entrusted to the child-welfare system and later as an adult sued the county social service agency for the negligence of social workers that kept Billy dependent and unfit to live in society.

On September 19, 1960, Billy and his 7-month-old sister were abandoned by their mother and found eating garbage behind a skid-row mission in Chicago. Billy's age (approximately 5) was unknown, and his speech was unintelligible. He was sent to an institution for the retarded in Michigan for 4 years. After a subsequent stormy foster-home placement, he was placed in Cook County's juvenile security prison for nearly 3 years, although the superintendent repeatedly petitioned the court to remove him.

In 1969, a legal aid lawyer, Pat Murphy, filed a class-action suit to release dependent and neglected children from prison on behalf of Billy. At 14, Billy was transferred to Elgin State Hospital, where he ran away ten times and was committed to the Illinois Security Hospital at Chester at the age of 18. Three years later Attorney Murphy intervened to enroll Nichols in a psychiatric program for 2 years, until he was jailed for car theft.

Lawsuits continue to attempt to redress the adverse impact of foster care. Class-action suits have been used to force improvements in child welfare services. In 1993, a class-action suit was filed by the American Civil Liberties Union and the Children's Rights Project, Inc., against Milwaukee County and the state of Wisconsin for failing to adequately protect children (WDCF n.d.). In response, the duties and authority of child welfare services were transferred from the county to a state Bureau of Milwaukee Child Welfare.

11.4   The Right to Be a Competent Parent

To say that a parent has a right to be competent might stretch the notion of rights too far. However, the logic for this right in our society is compelling and worth considering.

First of all, by definition the child-parent unit is irreducible. One half of the unit is a parent, and one half is a child. The interests of children and the interests of parents are inseparable, and both derive from a child's goal of responsible citizenship.

When parents face dangerous environments, poverty, unemployment, illness, or mental incapacities, their children inevitably face the same problems along with the risk of incompetent parenting. If children's interests are to be fulfilled, the interests of parents also must be taken into account. If children have a moral right to be competently parented, then parents have a moral right to be competent if they are not under the legal or physical custody of others.

A second reason is that the integrity of society itself depends upon competent parents. Incompetent parents threaten the stability of society and incur enormous public costs. Therefore, in this view becoming a competent parent deserves the status of a right.

Third, human beings have a genetic predisposition to parent competently in order to ensure the survival of our species. The goal of the reproductive cycle is parenthood, not just procreation. Conceiving and giving birth initiate parenthood as the fruition of the parents' own developmental stages of childhood, adolescence, and adulthood. In the most fundamental sense, competent parenthood fulfills the role of a woman or a man in the reproductive cycle. In order to preserve humanity and our society, adults have a right to fulfill their reproductive and parental potentials and for the state to help them become competent parents when possible.

11.5   Balancing the Rights of Parents and Minors

The essence of childhood at the beginning of the twentieth century was its dependency. Competent parents respected this dependency by judiciously exercising their authority. In the second half of the twentieth century, parental authority declined. As a result, childrearing has become a negotiation between parent and child with state and other agencies monitoring the process.

In the past, children were assumed to have capabilities we now rarely think they have because their labor was needed to help a family survive. In our efforts to give our children enjoyable childhoods, we tend to downplay their developmental need to assume responsibilities and obligations. Much confusion about adolescence is caused by stressful conflicts between adolescents' rights and their obligations to their parents. This highlights minors' responsibility to accept parental authority and to cooperate with their parents.

In some ways, the contemporary adolescent quest for independence represents a return to the time in which childhood did not extend beyond 14. The difference is that in earlier centuries persons were economically productive at the age of 14 and were not capable of reproduction, whereas now they have an increasing number of years beyond their fertility, often beyond adulthood, before they become economically productive.

The shift in power from adults to children and adolescents has emotional and economic repercussions. Parents may now look to their offspring for emotional support and give them excessive material goods that stress family finances. This shift includes the ability of children and adolescents to bring legal proceedings against their parents for alleged abuse without justification. All of this has eroded parental authority. This trend toward overindulgence is further abetted by the exploitation of adolescents as consumers.

Although our tradition of individual autonomy has largely kept government out of the family, the law is moving toward defining the limits of parental power. The Juvenile Justice and Delinquency Prevention Act of 1974 removed "status offenses" of incorrigibility and running away from juvenile delinquency. They are now regarded as related to inadequate or inappropriate parental authority rather than as acts stemming solely from the adolescents. The focus has shifted to therapeutic interventions.

When family matters are brought into the legal system, the interests of children, parents, and the state need to be carefully identified and balanced to determine the appropriate rule of law.

11.6 Valuing the Parental Rights of Competent Parents

If all parents and child-serving institutions served children's developmental interests, the issue of parental rights seldom would be raised.

Parental rights are no longer based on the juvenile ageist presumption that children are the property of their parents. Legal and physical custodial rights enable parents to discharge their responsibilities in the Parent-Society Contract (parenthood) that provides a strong moral imperative for public efforts to ensure children's safety and quality of life. Parental rights really are prerogatives essential for discharging the duties of parenthood.

A shift from the rights of parents to the best interests of children has gradually emerged in our courts. Parents who fail to meet specified conditions can have their parental rights terminated to permit adoption of a child. Most states have set aside the parental immunity doctrine so that children can sue their parents under certain circumstances.

We can balance the interests of children, parents, and the state if we truly value competent parents.

Political issues often revolve around conflicts between self-assertive social values associated with individual liberty and integrative cultural values that affirm the common good. Nowhere is this more evident than in attitudes toward parenthood (Table 11.1).

Table 11.1 Self-assertive social and integrative cultural values

Self-assertive social values	Integrative cultural values
Parental rights	Parental responsibilities
Passion (follow emotions)	Wisdom (reasoned thought)
Gratification now	Postponing gratification
Avoiding discomfort	Tolerating frustration
Freedom to make decisions	Capacity to make decisions
Reproductive liberty	Capacity to enter parenthood
Newborn baby as a parent's property	Newborn baby's right to a competent parent

11.7   Parents Need Family Resource Systems

As it now stands, the link between incompetent parents and social problems is obscured by other issues. Little public attention is devoted to the facts that parents can be held accountable to society through child labor, mandatory education, and child neglect and abuse laws. There is even less awareness that parenthood is a privilege that merits public monitoring and support because it is vital to the future of our nation.

The responsibilities of motherhood are better known than the responsibilities of fatherhood. As long as boys fail to postpone fatherhood until they are employed and men do not support their children, mothers and children will remain trapped in poor neighborhoods. Increasing the number of fathers involved in childcare means improved employment opportunities and workplace policies that include paternity leaves, flexible scheduling, employment-based childcare, and reasonable workloads. It means access to parent counseling to help couples manage disagreements and keep fathers involved. It means mentoring and community programs that model responsible fatherhood.

All of us depend upon the quantity and quality of other peoples' children. Our cultural values expect that even adults who are not parents must support the next generation. Support in return for service is an American rationale that combines individual freedom and the common good. Social Security and the post-World War II GI Bill are prime examples.

In the 1970s, most developed nations with the exception of the United States began to publicly support parents. They refused to accept, as Americans do, the risks posed by the inadequate care of babies and toddlers. These governments now protect children through paid parental leave for childbirth and sick childcare, regulated and subsidized childcare services, and flexible work hours. President Nixon vetoed the Comprehensive Child Development Act in 1971. Passed with bipartisan Congressional support, this Act would have provided parents similar support in the United States.

One consequence of that veto is that all states fell far short of meeting basic childcare requirements in 2005 according to the National Association of Child Care Resource & Referral Agencies (MMO 2008). Out of 150 possible points, the average state score was 70. Although Americans work much longer and more irregular hours

Table 11.2 Family resource system

Family resource system		
Parental responsibilities	Private resources	Public resources
Income	Self-employed	Dependent tax deductions
	Employment	Welfare-to-work payments
Health	Self-payment	Medical assistance
	Insurance or HMO	Social security insurance
Education	Private schools	Public schools
	Home schooling	School vouchers
Caregiving	Relative childcare	Subsidized childcare
	Home childcare	Tax deductions
	Center childcare	Welfare-to-work subsidies
	Workplace childcare	
Family stability	Grandparents	Family resource networks
	Private family services	Child protective services
	Friends and relatives	Temporary out-of-home care

than Europeans, we provide far less childcare and family leave. We would profit from adopting the support other developed countries offer parenthood.

In order to thrive, competent parents require family resource systems that include quality health care and education, a vital economy and low rates of unemployment, thriving urban centers and rural communities, safe neighborhoods, and a sense of common purpose underwritten by personal responsibility and accountability. As it now stands, families in the United States have access to some degree to family support systems that vary in the proportion of private and government funding. Our goal should be that these family support systems are able to meet the needs of all of our families (Table 11.2).

11.8   The United States Is Not a Family-Friendly Nation

Unfortunately, parenthood is not sufficiently recognized as a career in the United States that deserves public encouragement and support. Family-friendly social policies would go a long way toward removing the need to choose between unpaid parenthood and a paid career. If women were assured of childcare and economic assistance while pursuing higher education and career development during their childbearing years, fewer would delay child-bearing until later ages with all of its attendant risks and problems. For example, simple adjustments in college professors' tenure track policies would accommodate the childrearing responsibilities of faculty mothers and fathers.

Although individual parents have little power, local, state, and national organizations could recognize the service parents provide through their personal sacrifices and the resources they require for effectively pursuing the life-long career of parenthood.

11.9 The World That Ought to Be

Commercial marketing uses the world as it ought to be symbols. Slogans such as "Be all that you can be," "Reach out and touch someone," and "Own a piece of the rock" focus on appealing cultural values.

John Maynard Keynes concluded in the 1930s that unchecked "animal spirits" – emotions, human impulses, enthusiasms, and misperceptions – drive the economy into booms and busts in a market system that fails to govern itself (Barnett 2017). On the other hand, tempered by government and safely channeled into healthy capitalism, these same animal spirits can be a source of entrepreneurial energy and benefit everyone.

Most modern social and environmental problems like ill health, lack of community, violence, drugs, obesity, mental illness, long working hours, and large prison populations are more likely to occur in a society with large gaps between classes. Addressing inequality in our society would benefit everyone, the well-off as well as the poor.

Our young people's social, economic, health, and educational problems require integrative community and social efforts that include racial and cultural diversity. Still, our service systems often view children and youth separately from their families and communities. Programs for different categories of problems treat children as freestanding units and focus on school, peer, social class, racial, neighborhood, and societal factors rather than on their homes.

These problems could be minimized if our society recognized that parenthood is a career with economic and social value and that it is our society's foundation. This would shift the balance from self-centered consumerism to a friendlier and more integrative society.

Because competent parents are essential for our society's survival, minimum legal standards should be set for determining a person's readiness to assume these responsibilities.

11.9.1 Readiness for Parenthood

In most states, minors over 16 can obtain a marriage license with the consent of parents or guardians. Kansas and Massachusetts specify 12 for females and 14 for males. New Hampshire specifies 13 for females and 14 for males. If there is no parent or guardian, or if the guardian is an agency or department, consent can be given by a court. Marriage and military service can be regarded as acts of emancipation from minority status.

In contrast, most European nations make 18 the minimum age for marriage. In Malta, people may marry from the age of 16, although paradoxically the age of consent for sexual intercourse is 18. In Turkey, the legal age for marriage is 17 for girls and boys. In Ireland, a court can authorize the marriage of minors less than 18 under certain conditions.

Decisionmaking that leads to adolescent parenthood can be flawed and is an appropriate concern for public policy. In reality, immaturity renders a minor incapable of truly informed consent about marriage or becoming a parent. State laws governing marriage age and emancipation need to be updated to conform with the physical and psychological realities of adolescent development.

In spite of the rhetoric against adolescent pregnancies, our society does little to prepare parents for their new responsibilities. Dependent adult and young adolescent childbirths from unplanned and planned pregnancies are generally considered inevitable. These vulnerable parents, it is assumed, will somehow learn to handle parental responsibilities after the children are born.

Most of the literature about adolescent pregnancy and parenthood does not distinguish between minor and legally adult adolescents. Late adolescents 18- to 21-year-olds are usually considered adults.

Giving birth to a baby does not produce an adult brain or eliminate adolescent developmental issues. In a personal communication, John Mitchell, a developmental psychologist, called my attention to romanticized notions that can hide elementary facts:

> Romanticizing adolescence blinds us to the adolescent's capacity for life-diminishing choices. Romantics refuse to tally the teen suicides, runaways, juvenile sex trade, prisoners, broken mothers, damaged infants, and abusive fathers. In order to mature, the natural talent of youth must be aimed and trained.

Many adolescents are wishful thinkers who lack a future orientation because of their sense of invulnerability and their attraction to risk. They are easily swayed by the belief "it can't happen to me." This flavor "omniscient and omnipotent flavoring of adolescence" underlies the attitude "I don't care about that now" despite knowing that cigarettes, drugs, noise, and steroids produce diseases, addiction, and hearing loss while shortening lifespans. Babies and young children must be protected from these characteristics.

Adolescents who become pregnant have difficulty envisioning alternatives and reasoning through the consequences of childbirth. I had the following conversation with a 15-year-old white girl from a middle-class family:

Doctor: I'm told that the test results show that you are pregnant.
Patient: My boyfriend and I knew it because the condom broke.
Doctor: What do you plan to do?
Patient: I'm going to have my baby and keep it. My boyfriend will drop out of school to support us.
Doctor: Do you think that you are old enough to raise a child?
Patient: No. I certainly wouldn't try to get pregnant.
Doctor: Then how is it that you plan to raise this baby?
Patient: Oh, it was an accident. Besides, I don't like school, and I can get money to live on. I know a lot of kids who are doing it.

Adolescents who become pregnant are unprepared for the decisionmaking and responsibilities involved in parenthood. Mature adolescents recognize that they are not ready for parenthood and terminate their pregnancies or make an adoption plan.

11.9.2   Does the Biological Right to Procreate Extend to Persons of Any Age?

The progress of our society has been based on the rule of law, the tangible repository of our cultural values. We are able to transact business with checks and credit cards rather than cash because of the trust we have in the enforcement of our laws. Yet we are still reluctant to legislate standards for competent parenthood. The prime example is our failure to deal with the crisis of adolescent childbirth.

In the United States, there is a strong emphasis on reproductive freedom. The US Supreme Court described the right to procreate as a basic liberty in 1942 in Skinner v. Oklahoma. This has been interpreted as establishing the right to procreate. The political right might oppose the termination of any pregnancy and urge girls on to childbirth. The political left might hold that minor adolescents have the right to procreate when physically able to do so.

GirlMom.com describes itself as a "politically progressive, left-aligned, pro-choice, feminist" website that supports young mothers in their struggle for reproductive freedom and social support. It holds that "adolescents are socially conditioned to believe they are irresponsible. This creates a self-fulfilling prophecy in which adolescent parents believe they can't parent well and therefore don't." For GirlMom.com adolescent parenthood is not a crisis; the crisis is that adolescent parents do not receive enough public support.

Kristin Luker, a professor of sociology at the University of California-Berkeley, pointed out that adolescents have raised healthy children throughout human history (Luker 1997). She overlooked the fact that the average onset of menstruation has dropped from 16 to 12 years of age. She held that when good prenatal care and nutrition are available, the adolescent years are the best time to have babies from a physical point of view. Luker believes that "the jury is still out on whether or not adolescents make 'bad' parents."

This view conflicts with the moral and legal principle that a child is not the property of the genetic parent. From the moral point of view, parenthood is not a right awarded by procreation. As adoptive parents well know, it is earned by nurturing a child. From the legal point of view, genetic parents hold legal and physical custodian rights that are defined and can be revoked under child neglect and abuse laws. People who require legal and physical custodians themselves cannot be the legal and physical custodians of other persons...and newborn babies are other persons.

11.9.3   The Double Standard

Franklin Zimring, professor of law at the University of California-Berkeley, showed how accepting low-income adolescent parenthood while encouraging middle-class adolescents to terminate pregnancies or create adoption plans reveals a double standard (Zimring 2014). Ageism, sexism, and racism are all contributing factors as pointed out previously in this book.

Most adolescents who become pregnant realize that it is unwise to enter parenthood. But this wisdom often is not reinforced by their families, professionals, or society. To deprive adolescents of informed consent – the most important part of which is to ensure that they fully understand the responsibilities and consequences of parenthood – is an abrogation of parental and professional obligations. It violates the responsibility of professionals to do no harm.

Title XX of the Public Health Service Act specifies necessary services for Adolescent Family Life Demonstration Projects ([Title] 42 USC Chapter 6A). These include adoption counseling and referral services, education on the responsibilities of sexuality and parenting, and counseling for immediate and extended family members. This model should be available to all pregnant adolescents and their families as proposed in the next chapter.

11.9.4   Interests of Society

Our society generally regards preventing teen pregnancy as an important priority. Adolescent pregnancy does not stop being a social and personal crisis when a baby is born. Adolescent parenthood is an even greater crisis with additional health, welfare, and legal entanglements.

From society's point of view, should adolescent childbirth be approached reactively with damage control that might amplify its effects or thoughtfully with holistic planning that can dampen its effects? We have enough knowledge and opportunities to prevent damage if we connect adolescent parenthood to social problems. We do not need to feel helpless when an adolescent girl gives birth. We can apply the knowledge and problem-solving skills we already have.

Articulating cultural values that discourage premature sexual intercourse and parenthood can dramatically change adolescent behavior. Our country had success with this method in the early twentieth century, and the same success is evident in other countries today. The media's contemporary promotion of sexual behavior could be counteracted by a public health campaign highlighting the disadvantages of adolescent sexual intercourse and pregnancy just like those mounted against smoking, drug abuse, and drunk driving. Civic groups, churches, and celebrities could articulate standards for sexual behavior and parenthood just as they have to promote educational achievement. Mayor Michael Bloomberg initiated a teen pregnancy prevention campaign in New York City in March of 2013 (Office of the Mayor 2013). As might be expected, it stirred up criticism reflecting juvenile ageism that treats adolescent parents as adults and that ignores the right of newborn babies to have competent parents. Since then adolescent pregnancies have decreased significantly.

11.9.5 The Interests of Adolescents

Generally, a genetic parent is in the best position to raise a child. This principle guides family preservation in social work. It is affirmed by fetus-mother bonding throughout pregnancy and by breastfeeding after childbirth. But possessing the judgment, skills, and economic resources for parenthood is more important than the ability to conceive, give birth, and breastfeed. Genetic mothers and fathers who recognize they do not possess these qualities make adoption plans.

In 1983, Marie Winn called attention to children who were growing up without childhoods (Winn 1983). This is even more prevalent today. One symptom of the denigration of parenthood is the private and public support offered adolescent parents. It presumes that young people who cannot handle the responsibilities of their own lives can handle the responsibilities of parenthood despite our increasingly complicated world.

If we recognize adolescence as a developmental stage and if we define parenthood as an adult responsibility, we can restore childhood for children and adolescence for adolescents. Our society must realize that it cannot cut short the years of nurturing and protection its young need by allowing them to assume adult responsibilities prematurely in any venue.

We need to understand that the developmental characteristics of adolescence and the influences, or the lack thereof, of parents cause more adolescent pregnancies than ignorance and socioeconomic disadvantage. Antipoverty measures alone do not address parent-child relationships. In their Urban Institute article "A Mentor, Peer Group, Incentive Model for Helping Underclass Youth," Ronald Mincy and Susan Weiner (1990) noted that poverty is less important than the parents' behavior in influencing an adolescent girl's chance of becoming pregnant (Mincy and Wiener 1990).

Most importantly, we need to recognize that the charitable impulse to support adolescent parents can have unintended consequences. We need to shift from damage control to offering hope and empowerment.

State statutes use age grading to protect minors from activities beyond their abilities as well as to protect society from minor's inappropriate actions. Valuing parenthood enough to set a minimum standard could be a tipping point that shifts our society from self-assertive values to integrative cultural values. The most important issue facing us today is whether we value children and our nation's future enough to value parenthood as a career for adults who can handle its responsibilities.

11.9.6 Governmental Interventions in Family Life

If every citizen respected the rights of others, we would not need law enforcement. We would not need welfare if every individual was capable of, and had the opportunity to, lead an economically self-sufficient life. Unfortunately, everyone does not have these qualities or opportunities. We will always need law enforcement and some form of welfare.

We will always face the repercussions of incompetent parents if we do not set a standard for parenthood. Currently, all parents are assumed to be competent until they damage their children by neglect or abuse. A more accurate assumption is that the vast majority of parents are competent, but children and society need protection from the millions who are not.

We cannot assume competence in parenting any more than we can assume competence in any other activity that affects others. Licensing is intended to ensure that persons who do important things for others are competent and responsible. Irresponsible people conceive and bear children. For this reason, children and society now could have protection from incompetent parents by refining the prevention provisions of child neglect and abuse statutes. When parents are unable or unwilling to become competent, these statutes currently require that parental rights be terminated and the children be adopted.

Parents' abdication of their responsibilities necessitated laws that mandate parental participation in school conferences, the liability of grandparents for the children of their children, the liability of noncustodial parents for financial support, and the liability of parents for their children's actions. However, because of the subtle but powerful juvenile ageist assumption that children are the property of their parents – a belief concealed by the emphasis on family privacy and individual freedom – we intervene only after children have been significantly damaged by their parents.

If all parents were competent, the government would not need to be involved in family life. Because the neglect, abuse, and exploitation of children damage the next generation and create financial burdens for the present generation, the government has a clear-cut role in preventing neglect and abuse by setting standards for parenthood. All of us are paying an ever-larger share of the cost of rearing, educating, and treating children. Consequently, we all have a financial stake in preventing child neglect and abuse.

Around the world, governments are defining and regulating parenthood in response to conflicts between adult rights and children's needs. Underlying those conflicts is the erosion of the nuclear family. Children also are increasingly being viewed as commodities in the IVF and adoption marketplaces. A new paradigm is needed. The assumption that anyone regardless of age or capacity has legal and physical custodianship until a child is damaged must be challenged.

Our standards for responsible adulthood include supporting yourself legally and abiding by society's laws and regulations. Standards are set for foster parents, adoptive parents, divorce custody and visitation arrangements, childcare, preschools, schools, and others who are responsible for children's lives. A minimum standard for parenthood would protect children from neglect and abuse and all of us from the consequences. A standard will not create optimal childrearing scenarios but will identify the worst scenarios. What is good for children may be controversial, but what is bad for them is not as is clearly outlined in our child neglect and abuse laws.

Too many of our children are growing up in families that prevent them from becoming responsible, productive citizens. The repetitive cycle of adolescent and dependent adult parents followed by child abuse and neglect is the most preventable source of habitual crime and welfare dependency.

Our society needs a paradigm shift from our dominant self-assertive social values toward integrative cultural values. We can protect our nation's future by ensuring that all children have competent parents. We would then value parenthood as a career with as much economic and social value as paid employment. Parents would be able to compete economically with adults without children.

Because our society does not articulate expectations for parents, child neglect and abuse have reached epidemic proportions. Rates in the United States exceed that of all other developed nations. We only intervene after neglect and abuse have occurred, and often then ineffectively. Enormous public expenditures on treatment, rehabilitation, and incarceration result. This would change dramatically if our vision for America was that all our children will be raised by competent parents.

By failing to recognize newborn babies' right to competent parents with adequate resources, our society will continue to be anti-child and anti-parent. If we go on this way, we will ensure that America continues to decline. By addressing the basic needs of families, we can correct our course one child and one parent at a time. We need a system that sets a standard for parenthood and that includes in-home and community guidance for new parents along with ensuring that all families have adequate family resource systems.

11.9.7   What Do We Know?

Two vital aspects of parenthood are often overlooked. The first is that readiness for parenthood follows the adolescent stage of life. The ability to assume responsibility for one's own life is a prerequisite for assuming responsibility for the life of another person. The second is that parenthood is a developmental stage in life. Parents progress though egocentric, conventional, individualistic, and integrative phases of parenthood.

Controversies arise over whether pregnancy and childbirth themselves promote maturity, whether everyone has a right to parenthood regardless of age, and whether genetic parents are always the best persons to raise a child. In the past, preparation for parenthood occurred within families. With loosening family ties and family strife in the United States, preparation for parenthood now often must come from educational and clinical sources.

By entering parenthood, adolescents gain financial benefits in the form of Temporary Aid to Families with Dependent Children, Medicaid, counseling, educational accommodations, and childcare in addition to increased status with their peers and possibly families. Adoption is not appealing to them because it means parting with their babies and these benefits. Making an adoption plan also might evoke disapproval from relatives and peers. All these factors encourage adolescents to become parents despite the likelihood of unfavorable outcomes.

The best time for decisionmaking about parenthood and adoption plans is when a pregnancy first becomes known. The more mature adolescent parents are, the more likely they will choose not to enter parenthood. The overall evidence indicates that children who were adopted as babies fare as well as children reared in genetic families.

To ensure that children have competent parents, parenthood must be recognized as a developmental stage that follows adolescence and as an essential complement to childhood. Struggling parents also need access to collaborative systems of care, the topic of the next chapter.

References

Abrahamsen, D. (1952). *Who are the guilty? A study of education and crime.* New York: Grove Press.

Barnett, V. (2017). Keynes, animal spirits, and instinct: Reason plus intuition is better than rational. *Journal of the History of Economic Thought, 39*(3), 1–19.

Dwyer, J. G. (2009). Constitutional birthright: The state, parentage, and the rights of newborn persons. *Faculty Publications, 26.* http://scholarship.law.wm.edu/facpubs/26/. Accessed 6 July 2018.

Garbarino, J. (1995). *Raising children in a socially toxic environment.* San Francisco: Jossey-Bass.

Gorner, P. (1981, December 14). How Illinois turned its back on billy: A case of assault through neglect. *Chicago Tribune.*

Jill, S., Truesdell, J., Bailey, M. (2012). 20 years later: The boy who 'divorced' his parents. *People,* December 24. https://people.com/archive/20-years-later-the-boy-who-divorced-his-parents-vol-78-no-26/. Accessed 6 July 2018.

Luker, K. (1997). *Dubious conceptions: The politics of teenage pregnancy.* Cambridge, MA: Harvard University Press.

Mincy, R. B., & Wiener, S. J. (1990). *A mentor, peer group, incentive model for helping underclass youth* (Research paper). Washington, DC: The Urban Institute. https://eric.ed.gov/?id=ED337524. Accessed 6 July 2018.

MMO [The Mothers' Movement Online]. (2008). Leaving children to chance: NACCRRA's ranking of state standards and oversight of small family child care homes. http://www.mothersmovement.org/resources/childcare.htm. Accessed 6 July 2018.

Office of the Mayor, New York City. (2013). Mayor Bloomberg discusses city's new teen pregnancy prevention campaign in weekly radio address. http://www1.nyc.gov/office-of-the-mayor/news/081-13/mayor-bloomberg-city-s-new-teen-pregnancy-prevention-campaign-weekly-radio-address. Accessed 6 July 2018.

Parentage Act. (2017). The National Conference of Commissioners on Uniform State Laws. http://www.uniformlaws.org/Act.aspx?title=Parentage%20Act%20(2017). Accessed 6 July 2018.

Shanley, M. L. (2001). *Making babies, making families.* Boston: Beacon Press.

Smith v. Alameda County Social Services Agency. (1979). Decided: March 23, 1979. https://caselaw.findlaw.com/ca-court-of-appeal/1835333.html. Accessed 6 July 2018.

[Title] 42 USC Chapter 6A, Subchapter XVIII: Adolescent Family Life Demonstration Projects. From title 42—The public health and welfare, Chapter 6A—public health service. http://uscode.house.gov/view.xhtml?path=/prelim@title42/chapter6A/subchapter18&edition=prelim. Accessed 6 July 2018.

Volunteers of America. (2018). Through the eyes of a child: Life with a mother in prison. https://www.voa.org/pdf_files/life-with-a-mother-in-prison. Accessed 6 July 2018.

Vopat, M. C. (2015). *Children's rights and moral parenting.* New York: Lexington Books.

WDCF [Wisconsin Department of Children and Families]. (n.d.). Milwaukee County Child Protective Services (MCPS) Children's Rights Lawsuit. https://dcf.wisconsin.gov/mcps/childrensrights. Accessed 6 July 2018.

Westman, J. C. (2007). *Licensing parents: Can we prevent child abuse and neglect?* Da Capo Press (ebook). ASIN: B00A4JN9SW. Boston, MA.

Winn, M. (1983, May 18). The loss of childhood. *The New York Times*. https://www.nytimes.com/1983/05/08/magazine/the-loss-of-childhood.html. Accessed 6 July 2018.

Zimring, F. E. (2014). *The changing world of adolescence*. New Orleans: Quid Pro Books.

Chapter 12
Overcoming Our Crisis-Recoil Response

*The most important measure of any society is not the standard
that its strongest members set for themselves, but rather where
they fix the moral bar for the weaker.*

Kay S. Hymowitz (2006)

Anthropologist Margaret Mead eloquently called attention to the damaging institutional response to children when they are treated as independent persons during crises (Brazelton 1984). Since most crisis interventions occur after rather than before damage occurs, children frequently are victims of crisis-recoil responses in which an overreaction to crises in their lives is followed by recoiling from the causes of the crises.

12.1 Crisis-Recoil Political Response

Our crisis-recoil political system overreacts to crises and then ignores their causes. This avoids responsibility for making difficult decisions. As a result, there is little or no emphasis on prevention or concern about the future impact of current actions. Because of our crisis-recoil political response, we react to child neglect and abuse without addressing their underlying causes.

This is seen when children are removed from their homes during a crisis as if they were independent persons rather than recognizing their dependence on their parents. This response often includes little to strengthen their families. Later, the inevitable shortage of foster homes is dealt with by seeking more foster homes and raising reimbursement for them rather than by addressing the family problems that necessitated so many foster homes in the first place.

Public policies fail to recognize that a child is half of a two-person unit that depends on the integrity of the mediating structures of family, neighborhood, school, and community. Child protective services only intervene when children show evidence of

© Springer Nature Switzerland AG 2019
J. C. Westman, *Dealing with Child Abuse and Neglect as Public Health
Problems*, https://doi.org/10.1007/978-3-030-05897-5_12

serious damage from abuse and/or neglect. As a result, services that focus on individual children and that fragment families have been overdeveloped, while resources that support parenthood and community building have been underdeveloped. Shirley Johnson's family described in Chap. 1 of this book is a typical example.

Another obvious example is our response to and punishment of criminal behavior. Police intervene after crimes have been committed, and more prisons are built in the belief that the penal system will solve the social problem of crime. Punishment of crime becomes a reality-avoidance mechanism that recoils from the underlying causes. Punishment of a culprit permits the public to believe that the crisis created by a crime has been resolved.

The crisis-recoil phenomenon is illustrated further by regulations that mandate medical treatment for grossly defective newborns. The response to the crisis at birth is to save the child's life. Recoil from the cause of the newborn's crisis and its repercussions means there is no assessment of the impact of preserving the newborn's life and no provision for treatment after the child leaves the intensive-care neonatal unit. The child remains dependent on expensive technology to maintain physical life too often with the disruption and potential financial ruin of the family.

The lack of appreciation of the importance of family ties also is highlighted in the crisis-recoil management of divorce custody and visitation matters. After the crisis of divorce has subsided, the lack of access to their children makes parents aware of how important their children are to them. They recoil through custody contests that usually are harmful to their children.

The crisis-recoil nature of our political and human services systems only aggravates our social problems. We need to strengthen the mediating structures that can solve those problems by more clearly articulating cultural values that support family, neighborhood, and community relationships. We can do this by applying the basic principles of public health.

12.2   Three Kinds of Prevention of Social Problems

The public health concepts of primary, secondary, and tertiary prevention can be profitably applied to our social problems, especially child abuse and neglect. Primary prevention is the prevention of a disease or harm. Secondary prevention treats a disease or harm. Tertiary prevention manages and minimizes disability from the disease or harm. As it stands now, our social, educational, and mental health services are oriented largely to secondary and tertiary prevention.

12.2.1   Primary Prevention

Home visitation programs for the parents of newborns are available in many communities. They offer both prenatal and natal services designed to strengthen families on both a request and referral basis. Healthy Families America is an example of a nationally recognized evidence-based home visiting program model designed to work with overburdened families who are at risk for adverse childhood experiences, including child maltreatment.

The premier neighborhood organization Harlem Children's Zone, Inc. (HCZ) began in 1970 as Rheedlen (HCZ 1990). HCZ worked with young children and their families as the city's first truancy-prevention program. In the early 1990s, it ran a pilot project that brought a range of support services to a single block. The idea was to address all the problems that disadvantaged families faced from crumbling apartments to failing schools and from violent crime to chronic health problems. In 1997, the agency began a network of programs for a 24-block area. In 2007, the Zone Project grew to almost 100 blocks. Today the HCZ serves more than 8000 children and 6000 adults.

In North Carolina, the East Durham Children's Initiative (EDCI n.d.) is an example of efforts around the country to replicate the Harlem Children's Zone. In Omaha, Nebraska, Building Bright Futures sponsors school-based health centers and offers mentoring and enrichment services.

Our public health system is devoted to preventing physical, mental, and social disorders. The system promotes education, advocacy, services, and enforcement guided by legislation. In addition, the Child Abuse Prevention and Treatment Act of 1974 placed the moral weight of the federal government behind professional interventions to help struggling families (ECSO n.d.).

As public health knowledge about preventable conditions emerges, legislation is enacted. Examples include mandated immunization of school children and testing at birth for phenylketonuria, a treatable predisposition to mental and neurological disorders. The Keeping Children and Families Safe Act of 2003 requires states to ensure that health-care providers report babies affected by prenatal drug exposure to child protective services (NLIHC 2018).

Many states have gone further. Physicians originally in New Jersey and now in other states are required to educate expectant mothers about postpartum depression and screen new mothers for it (Postpartum Support International n.d.). HIV testing of pregnant women is mandatory in some states because protecting the unborn child supersedes the mother's right to refuse testing. These measures are precedents for legislation on the crisis of adolescent childbirth.

The international response to the H1N1 flu epidemic of 2009 illustrates how national leadership can galvanize action when we know the nature of a problem and what to do about. Modern public health, which quickly recognizes changes in the course of an illness and pours out resources to prevent it, shows our ability to plan and take action when we decide to do so.

A flu epidemic is far less important to our nation's wellbeing and our leadership in the world economy than the birth of babies who are destined to fail in life and cause the majority of our social problems. We know what the problem is and what to do about it, but we lack the national leadership and the political will to apply what we know and to act.

Health care underwent a paradigm shift when our focus on treating the disabilities caused by poliomyelitis shifted to preventing polio through immunization.

Dentistry underwent a paradigm shift when it shifted the focus from treating dental caries to preventing it through fluoridation of our water supply.

Human services are beginning a paradigm shift from protecting children by removing them from their homes to strengthening their families. Unfortunately, the next paradigm shift to ensuring that newborns have competent parents is obstructed by juvenile ageism that objects to government invasion of the privacy of families and restriction of the freedom of parents to do as they wish with their children. As a result, we ignore newborns' most basic need for parents who can provide adequate care for them and do not enact the legislation needed to fill that need.

12.2.2   Secondary Prevention

Current child welfare interventions focus on secondary prevention with dependent parents. The hope is that they will not neglect or abuse their babies and that subsequent births will be prevented. The emphasis needs to be shifted to the primary prevention of dependent parenthood. Child neglect and abuse statutes already allow termination of parental rights at childbirth when circumstances warrant, including the absence of a competent parent. These statutes can specifically address the unavailability of a qualified legal and physical custodian. In order to function effectively, child welfare workers need this kind of support from legislation.

The Strengthening Families Program was developed in the early 1980s by Karol Kumpfer (Strengthening Families Foundation n.d.). Its 14 sessions cover child development, behavior management, child skills training, family skills enhancement and attachment bonding, and psychoeducational material targeted at improving the child-parent relationship. Currently, it is being used with struggling families in every state and in 17 nations. It results in higher rates of family reunification than traditional methods.

12.2.3   Tertiary Prevention

Tertiary prevention aims to reduce the damage incurred from child abuse and neglect. Collaborative Systems of Care provide integrated support and resources for struggling families in a collaborative, family-centered way that leads to better outcomes for individuals, families, and communities (CSC 2018). They also reduce duplication of effort and are an effective use of limited resources.

Wraparound/Coordinated Services Teams emerged in the early 1980s as a collaborative planning approach to community-based care for children and youth with complex mental health and related challenges. These teams are promoted and monitored by the National Wraparound Initiative (NWIC 2018). A Wraparound Team brings together family members, service and resource providers, and people from the family's social support network. Team members create, implement, and monitor a plan to meet family needs.

Wraparound planning focuses on meeting the needs and reaching the goals that family members identify as most essential. The Wraparound process is individualized, culturally competent, strength based, and outcome oriented.

Each Wraparound site has a coordinating committee made up of parents and representatives from agencies and organizations that serve children and families. The committee's responsibilities include:

- Developing policies and procedures, including an interagency service agreement
- Developing and implementing a plan for sustainability
- Evaluation and quality assurance, including family and provider satisfaction

Wraparound teams have four phases of involvement: (1) strengths and needs assessment; (2) an individualized plan of care based on identified strengths and needs, including crisis response plans for home, school, and community; (3) ongoing monitoring of the plan with the support of team members; and (4) plans for transition from the formal team process to ensure the family has a voice in decisions, access to resources, and ownership of their achievements.

Multisystemic Therapy (MST) is an intensive family-community-based treatment program that focuses on the world of chronic and violent juvenile offenders—their homes, schools, and neighborhoods (MST n.d.). MST works with adolescents between the ages of 12 and 17 who have arrest histories. The MST team of several therapists is intensively involved with families through at least three home visits a week and is available by telephone 24/7 for 11–30 weeks. MST has been applied in the United States and at least seven other countries.

12.3 Governmental Power Versus Individual Rights

For good reason, we restrict the government's power to intervene in private lives to circumstances in which serious harm to others or society is likely. When people abuse their freedom to act, the challenge is to identify situations that warrant legal intervention. The freedom to procreate and raise children is among our most cherished rights. Any limitation of this right will understandably prove to be controversial. Nonetheless, our laws clearly state that parents are not free to neglect or abuse their children.

In Carey v. Population Services International in 1977, the US Supreme Court noted "the incidence of sexual activity among minors is high, and the consequences of such activity are frequently devastating...." (Cornell Law School Legal Information Institute (LII) n.d.). This recognition—especially when minors already have limited legal privileges—opens the door to an in loco parentis role for the state whenever a dependent minor chooses to continue a pregnancy to childbirth.

In legal terms, being a minor is a disability. The gradual achievement of adult independence is the process of outgrowing the disability of infancy. Our age-grading laws recognize that adolescents are incapable of making life-altering decisions. Progressively awarding adult privileges protects a youth's healthy development and safety.

Driver training and graduated licensing programs, for example, significantly reduce fatalities among young drivers. The proposed Safe Teen and Novice Driver Uniform Protection Act of 2011 (H.R. 1515) would create a National Graduated Driver licensing law that limits night driving, reduces in-car distractions, puts a cap on the number of friends in the car, and increases the required hours of training and supervision (H.R. 1515). This kind of age-grading principle should apply to parenthood as well. This federal Act was not adopted in 2011 or 2012 on the grounds that it is a state issue.

Unfortunately, legal traditions have followed outdated common law that fails to recognize adolescence as a developmental stage. Adolescent immaturity is ignored when parental rights and legal emancipation are granted to minors. These traditions both view adolescence as a temporary status rather than a stage of development.

Often adolescent parents need double protection from their own incompetence as parents as well as from that of their parents. The first weeks and months of a baby's life are crucial periods that have profound and lasting consequences. Their babies need protection from their young parents as well as from their extended family. To ensure that both adolescents and their babies receive competent parenting, we need a more realistic way to view the legal status of the babies of adolescent parents.

12.4 Newborns Need Competent Custodians

At the beginning and possibly at the end of life, a human being requires a legal and physical custodian or guardian. When the elderly are no longer competent to make decisions and manage their own lives, states enable relatives to take over as conservators for their finances and health care. We have no problem accepting the need for state involvement in the affairs of incompetent adults. We do have difficulty accepting the same need at the beginning of life when state involvement is even more critical. The future holds newborn persons' entire lives, not their deaths.

Fortunately, when the rights of children and parents conflict, the evolving legal trend is to place children's "best interests" first. A baby's interests rise above the wishes of her or his dependent parents and their families. In fact, the babies of dependent minors and adults do not have legal and physical custodians capable of:

- Ensuring they receive nurturance and life's material necessities
- Making prudent decisions concerning their welfare and wellbeing
- Arranging for and authorizing health care
- Advocating their interests

In some states, antiquated laws regard childbirth as an act that emancipates minors from their parents' authority. Nevertheless, minors cannot be legal and physical custodians of their babies, a reality recognized whenever a court appoints a guardian ad litem (an officer of the court) to represent a minor parent in adoption proceedings. Simply put, minors cannot be legal and physical custodians of other persons because they require legal and physical custodians themselves.

The age-grading principle built into our laws prevents minors from assuming responsibility for the life of another person. Their brain development and their emotional and social maturity do not enable them to make decisions that permanently affect their own lives let alone those of their babies.

Right now, grandparents can have statutory financial liability for a grandchild's support but not legal or physical custodianship. They and other supportive family members need to be released from this trap. Some states now permit de facto custodianship when minor parents default on the care of their children to adult relatives, but this is too little, too late.

The adolescent childbirth crisis now evokes a number of interventions ranging from paternity determination to group home placement for mother and baby. These interventions often span months or years while the baby's interests are neglected. We must view adolescent childbirth from the newborn baby's point of view. We need a vision in which the birth of every baby is a cause for celebration of a new citizen's opportunity to succeed in our nation.

When it is clear that this will not be the case, we need to bring a baby's birth as close as possible to this vision. Because adolescent childbirth is a public health crisis masked by powerful emotions, we need to use existing health, social welfare, and legal resources when a minor's pregnancy is first identified. We also need to establish best practices to ensure that an unborn baby's interests come first. To reach this goal, we can start by implementing the primary prevention provisions of our child neglect and abuse statutes that apply to newborns who will not have a qualified parent…a legal and physical custodian. As has been made clear, the newborn babies of dependent persons do not have qualified legal and physical custodians.

The present stance of intervening only after children are damaged is inhumane and costly. This can be remedied by mandating Parenthood Planning Counseling for all pregnant minors and dependent adults that include their custodians. We need to craft legal and clinical procedures to deal with the fact that both adolescent mothers and fathers and their babies require protection. Resolving critical parenthood issues before birth is the single most important step we can take to reduce crime and welfare dependency in our nation.

12.4.1 Parenthood Planning Counseling

Health-care professionals are key to Parenthood Planning Counseling for pregnant girls, dependent women, dependent fathers, and their families. As mentioned before, Title XX of the Public Health Service Act already requires that Adolescent Family

Life Demonstration Projects offer this kind of counseling that includes the minor's family to address the option of adoption and the responsibilities of sexuality and parenting. In this context, the following programs can offer or arrange for parenthood planning counseling:

- Family planning and health-care clinics that provide pregnancy diagnosis
- Medicaid Prenatal Care Coordination services
- Prenatal care clinics
- Prenatal home visitation programs

Within these programs, professionals can approach dependent pregnant mothers and their families with open minds. The goal is to develop a shared understanding of concerns, priorities, strengths, and challenges, always with sensitivity to cultural factors. To this end, materials are available to assist counseling with Black, Latino, American Indian, and Southeastern Asian families, such as provided by the Center for the Improvement of Child Caring (CICC n.d.).

When it occurs, pregnancy usually represents the first life-altering decision of a girl's life. She and the baby's father when involved can be expected to be uncertain about what to do. Most adolescents have little if any counseling about their options in managing their pregnancies. Along with facts and reassurance, they need help exploring their fantasies, fears, anxieties, guilt, and hopes. The adolescent's parents might express their guilt through anger toward or support of the pregnant girl and the father. All parties need to explore their feelings about the pregnancy.

It is important to know that many girls embrace pregnancy to avoid isolation and loneliness. Many fear facing their feelings of emptiness and inadequacy and seek the love of a baby. Abandonment by their fathers often accentuates these feelings. The resulting feelings of despair and unworthiness can result in unwise decisions.

Ideally decisions regarding the course of a pregnancy should be made when the pregnancy is diagnosed, and its existence is accepted by all concerned. This is the most clearheaded time to consider everyone's interests…those of the unborn child, mother, father, their families, and society.

Discovering a pregnancy is an emotional event. Still, the physical and emotional changes of advanced pregnancy and childbirth have not yet occurred. The potential mother and father and their families, therefore, are in the best position to fully weigh the pros and cons of each possible course. If the decision is to continue the pregnancy, the interests of the newborn baby should move to the forefront. This provides 5–7 months to work through guilt, shame, pride, and fantasies about childrearing… and to plan for adoption at birth if that is the best course.

If a decision is postponed, the hormonal and physical changes of late pregnancy cloud objective thinking. After childbirth, prolactin and oxytocin activate instincts that motivate mothers to strongly attach to their babies. Pitressin (vasopressin) produces similar responses in fathers. This is the time when objective decision-making is the least likely to occur.

Consummating the decision-making process during pregnancy also is critical for the wellbeing of the newborn. The first weeks and months of a baby's life have profound developmental consequences, especially for the attachment bonding process. The compelling interests of the newborn should take precedence over the traditional view that mothers and fathers need time after birth to decide about adoption.

12.4.2 Parenthood Planning Teams

The existing prevention provisions of child neglect and abuse statutes are the basis for Parenthood Planning Counseling through Parenthood Planning Teams. Public health practices like case reporting, counseling, and law enforcement can be used to implement counseling for all adolescent parents. Currently, these interventions are mandated only in cases where child neglect or abuse is suspected.

A Parenthood Planning Team would, depending on individual circumstances, consist of two or more of the following: a family planning counselor, prenatal care counselor or public health nurse, a child welfare worker to implement the guardianship petition process, other professionals involved with the adolescent or her family, and, when appropriate, a guardian ad litem. The potential for this kind of teamwork exists now in prenatal home visitation, prenatal care coordination, and Wraparound/Coordinated Services Teams.

A Parenthood Planning Team would be activated whenever childbirth is on the horizon for minors or adults with developmental disabilities, previous termination of parental rights, or incarceration as violent felons or domestic abusers. These categories need to be considered individually with a focus on the interests of everyone involved.

In addition, the criteria for incarceration need to be revised. Most of the 84,000 women in federal and state prisons are serving a year or less for possession or trafficking in illegal substances, shoplifting, bad checks, or stolen credit cards. Of those in Illinois, for example, most are in their 30s with three or four children, 63% are high school dropouts, 60% have substance abuse problems, 85% are single mothers, and most are victims of domestic abuse. We need to shift their sentencing from incarceration to community management so that their families are not disrupted. Then they can receive the help they need through Collaborative Systems of Care, such as Wraparound/Coordinated Services Teams.

We need to consider the life circumstances and abilities of each parent in order to identify the most appropriate options. Because each parent's situation is unique, a Parenthood Planning Team would determine the most appropriate course of action. Just as a patient's capacity to give informed consent for health care must be evaluated, the team must evaluate a minor parent's decision-making capacities for entering parenthood.

12.4.3   Short-Term Desires and Long-Term Interests

Most of us understand that we should eat reasonably, live within our means, avoid addictions, be sexually responsible, keep promises, and hold undesirable impulses in check. Yet, we regularly violate at least some of these tenets … not because we want to harm ourselves but because we fail to control our urges. Most importantly, pop culture often glorifies self-indulgent and self-defeating actions … "just do it."

In this ambivalent social atmosphere, pregnant girls, conceiving boys, and dependent adults need Parenthood Planning Counseling along with their parents. This counseling is vital for making decisions that place the interests of the newborn baby first followed by those of the adolescents, their families, and society.

Such counseling should not be based on either supporting the status quo or satisfying individual desires. It should be focused on the aim of productive citizenship for adolescents and dependent adults as well as for their newborn babies. It places long-term interests ahead of short-term impulses.

Most adolescents and dependent adults who become pregnant have difficulty envisioning the alternatives and consequences. They need guidance in identifying their babies' and their own self-interests along with the consequences of their choices. They need to understand the responsibilities of parenthood. They need to fully realize that a baby is not a possession but a human being entitled to competent parenting. They need to fully realize the impact of imposing the burdens of child-drearing on their parents and relatives. They need to realistically understand adoption.

Young people also need help understanding that adolescence is an important life stage that will be shortchanged by parenthood's physical, emotional, psychological, and economic consequences. A girl needs to understand that parenthood exposes her and her child to elevated risks of poverty, inadequate education, depression, welfare dependency, and prison. Even with financial benefits, parenthood will not eliminate disadvantaged circumstances.

We need to create opportunities and language for sharing our knowledge about the best interests of a child so that young people can make these life-altering decisions.

12.5   The Decision-Making Process

In order to seriously consider whether or not to enter parenthood, a girl needs help choosing the most advantageous course. She needs to understand that her baby is not her possession and is a human being with a separate life. She needs help envisioning her future and the future of her baby. Then, she can distinguish her self-interests from her baby's interests. She can see that parenthood would deprive her and her baby of vital opportunities. She can see that her parental responsibility can be fulfilled by ensuring that her baby has a family that can provide a fulfilling life.

Choosing not to enter parenthood and to make an adoption plan allows young people to develop as responsible, caring individuals. They realize they are not ready to enter parenthood. They know they can compensate for past mistakes by not making another. They can act in the best interests of their babies, the innocent parties. They mature by planning ahead and making painful decisions. They gain satisfaction from mastering a confusing emotional crisis. They heal painful feelings by creating a better future for themselves and their babies. Sixteen-year-old Stephanie chose to make an adoption plan:

> I'm not a selfish person.... A selfish person would have wanted to tough it out with her child and end up on welfare.... The only thing I could give my child is love. I couldn't give her all that she needs. A mother who really loves her baby puts her up for adoption. I'm not going on welfare just to raise my child.

The sacrifice and altruism involved in adoption enable genetic mothers to see themselves as mature persons whose decisions serve their own and their babies' interests.

References

Brazelton, T. B. (1984). *The growing child in family and society: An interdisciplinary study in parent-infant bonding.* Tokyo: University of Tokyo Press.

CICC [Center for the Improvement of Child Caring]. (n.d.). http://www.ciccparenting.org/. Accessed 6 July 2018.

Cornell Law School Legal Information Institute (LII). (n.d.). Carey v. Population Services International. https://www.law.cornell.edu/supremecourt/text/431/678#ZO-431_US_678n20. Accessed 19 Oct 2018.

CSC [Collaborative Systems of Care]. (2018). The coordinated services team initiative collaborative systems of care resources. http://www.wicollaborative.org/. Accessed 6 July 2018.

ECSO [Early Childhood Services of Omaha, Nebraska]. http://www.ecsomaha.org/bbf.html. Accessed 6 July 2018.

EDCI [East Durham Children's Initiative]. http://edci.org/en. Accessed 6 July 2018.

Hymowitz, K. S. (2006). *Marriage and caste in America: Separate and unequal families in a post-marital age.* New York: Ivan R. Dee.

MST Services. http://www.mstservices.com/. Accessed 6 July 2018.

NLIHC [National Low Income Housing Coalition]. (2018). 40 years ago: Child abuse prevention and treatment act passed. http://nlihc.org/article/40-years-ago-child-abuse-prevention-and-treatment-act-passed. Accessed 6 July 2018.

NWIC [The National Wraparound Implementation Center]. (2018). http://www.nwic.org/. Accessed 6 July 2018.

Postpartum Support International. Information about National and State Legislative action related to perinatal mood disorders and maternal mental health. http://www.postpartum.net/professionals/legislation/. Accessed 6 July 2018.

Strengthening Families Foundation. The strengthening families program. https://www.strengtheningfamiliesprogram.org/. Accessed 6 July 2018.

Chapter 13
The Parent-Society Contract

> *We hold these truths to be self-evident, that all men are created equal, that they are endowed by their Creator with certain unalienable Rights, that among these are Life, Liberty and the pursuit of Happiness.*
>
> Declaration of Independence of the United States of America
>
> *We the People of the United States, in Order to form a more perfect Union, establish Justice, insure domestic Tranquility, provide for the common defence, promote the general Welfare, and secure the Blessings of Liberty to ourselves and our Posterity, do ordain and establish this Constitution for the United States of America.*
>
> The United States Constitution

The United States was founded with the dedication to provide an opportunity for everyone to succeed in life through an implicit Parenthood-Society Contract. Our usual interpretations of our two founding documents acknowledge that the reference to "men" actually means men and women, but we do not think of "unalienable Rights" as including children, especially newborn babies. We also overlook the phrase "secure the Blessings of Liberty to ourselves and our *Posterity.*"

In one sense, it is appropriate to exclude minors from liberties and responsibilities that are within the purview of adulthood. It also is important to recognize that "the pursuit of Happiness" actually refers to the opportunity to flourish in life, not to just pursue pleasure. Still, the Declaration of Independence does include all human beings regardless of age, and the Constitution does explicitly refer to "our Posterity"—succeeding generations, which means our children. These commitments boil down to the right in the United States of every newborn baby to have an opportunity to flourish in life.

In the past, children have been treated as the personal property of their parents. Under Roman law, the patria potestas doctrine gave fathers life and death power over their children. To this day, the popular presumption is that children are the possessions of their parents.

© Springer Nature Switzerland AG 2019
J. C. Westman, *Dealing with Child Abuse and Neglect as Public Health Problems*, https://doi.org/10.1007/978-3-030-05897-5_13

In contrast, since the Enlightenment of the eighteenth century, parenthood in Western cultures has been seen as a contract between parents and society by philosophers and by evolving legal codes. Parents are awarded rights by society in exchange for discharging their responsibilities.

John Locke and William Blackstone held that parental rights and powers arise from their duty to care for their offspring. Both held that, if a choice is forced upon society, it is more important to protect the rights of children than to protect the rights of adults (Epstein 1998).

Americans instinctively respect the family as an institution that helps facilitate all other aspects of life. The family fosters attachments across generations, provides a nurturing environment in which to raise children, and is a means of transmitting values from one generation to the next. It is the foundation of our society and as such requires its support and monitoring. Monitoring of families takes place now in the United States through the legal *parens patriae* ("parent of the people") doctrine that draws upon the *Declaration of Independence* and the Constitution and employs the inherent power and authority of the state to protect people who are legally unable to act on their own behalf. It gives state courts the ultimate power to terminate parental rights and is based on four presumptions:

- Children do not choose the families into which they are born.
- Childhood and adolescence are periods of dependency and require supervision.
- The family is of primary importance, but the state should play a role in a child's education and intervene when parents fail to carry out their responsibilities.
- When parents disagree or fail to exercise their authority, the appropriate authority to determine a child's or an adolescent's interests is a public official.

The *parens patriae* doctrine empowers the state to compel parents and minors to act in ways that are beneficial to society. It never meant that the state would assume parenting functions. Instead, the state is responsible for protecting the best interests of children under the guidance of two principles:

- The wellbeing of society depends upon children being raised by parents who are willing and able to fulfill the responsibilities of parenthood.
- These responsibilities of parenthood are defined by child neglect and abuse statutes.

In practice, our national, state, county, and urban governments currently recognize the Parenthood-Society Contract and their responsibilities for "our Posterity." They support families raising children in a number of ways, including providing public assistance, public education, community resources, recreational facilities, and tax preferences. As a society, however, we need to do more than merely provide benefits. We need to ensure that parents and prospective parents fully comprehend the responsibilities of parenthood. We need to do a better job of ensuring that they possess the capacities and resources needed to meet those responsibilities. In short, we need to expect greater accountability on the part of parents.

The ability to conceive or to give birth says nothing about a parent's ability or willingness to be a responsible parent. We need, therefore, to set a minimum standard for parenthood based on our cultural expectation embodied in the Parenthood-Society Contract that all citizens, including newborn babies, will have an opportunity to succeed in life. By producing our nation's Posterity—our future citizens—parents implicitly enter the Parenthood-Society Contract in which they are expected to raise their children to become productive citizens in return for society's support in providing resources and environments suitable for childrearing.

Because the Parenthood-Society Contract is not openly recognized and honored on both sides, we now have too many parents who are unwilling or unable to raise their children successfully. Even more importantly, as a society we fall short of providing the reliable resources and environments parents need to raise their children. We too often rely upon uncoordinated professions and social services to intervene long after social problems arise and in ways that cannot deal with the underlying causes of intergenerational poverty, crime, and welfare dependency. Moreover, these unconnected, crisis-recoil responses to problems generally do not apply practices that we know work to prevent problems in the first place. If this fragmented approach was applied to public health, we would immunize only a fraction of our population and then treat only a fraction of the individuals who became infected and many of them too late to do much good. The result would be pandemics of diseases analogous to what we now see with our widespread educational failures, endemic crime, and welfare dependency.

Our failure to expect more from the parents who raise our nation's children—to hold them more accountable—has disastrous consequences, including the following (Lepore 2016):

- Three million children are referred to child protective services every year.
- Eleven million children have been seriously damaged by abuse and/or neglect.
- Millions of children fall into the Cradle to Prison/Welfare-Dependency Pipeline and experience disastrous outcomes in life.

For humanitarian and financial reasons…for our nation's prosperity…we must try to remove government from direct involvement in family lives by preventing the formation of, and reducing the number of, families that spawn our social problems. We need a paradigm that protects everyone's interests when a baby is born. This is especially the case with adolescent parents. Births to adolescents should evoke full consideration first of the interests of the babies, then of the adolescents, then of their relatives, and ultimately of society. There is a minimum standard for the adoption of animals. The American Humane Association employs an interview process to ensure that each animal adopted is matched to the most compatible new owner. The applicant must be 18 years of age or older and able to provide for the pet's needs.

As a society, we have not carefully thought through how to protect everyone's interests. As a result, our responses are reactive rather than proactive. We automatically shift from advocating teen pregnancy prevention, such as the efficacious Colorado Family Planning Initiative (CDPHE 2018), to supporting adolescent parents based on our perceived lack of alternatives. In fact, the reasons for preventing teen pregnancy do not disappear when a teenager becomes pregnant. Adolescent childbirth is an even greater public health crisis than adolescent pregnancy. Focusing only on the adolescent ignores the interests of the baby. Focusing only on the baby ignores the interests of the adolescent. In both situations, the interests of the family and society usually are ignored. It is ironic indeed that the American Humane Association restricts animal adoptions to adults, while we automatically accord full parental rights to minors. The paradigm we need also would apply to childbirth by adults with legal guardians themselves and by adults who courts have determined to be unfit parents.

13.1   Preventing Undesirable Lifestyles

For all of these dependent parents, parenthood is an undesirable lifestyle. As a society, we actively try to prevent undesirable lifestyles. We devote public resources to preventing domestic violence, child neglect and abuse, drug abuse, alcoholism, smoking, obesity, sexually transmitted diseases, and adolescent pregnancy. When individuals persist in such behaviors despite interventions, we take one of two courses:

- When harm involves only the individual, we care for them. For example, our health-care systems help both smokers and nonsmokers.
- When behavior harms others, as with sexually transmitted diseases, public health and law enforcement systems intervene. Adolescent and dependent adult parenthood has repercussions far beyond the parents. Its short- and long-term effects harm their babies, their families, and our society. A possible paradigm for protecting the interests of all parties at childbirth would be to set a minimum standard for parenthood.

References

CDPHE [Colorado Department of Public Health and Environment]. (2018). Report: Taking the unintended out of pregnancy: Colorado's success with Long-Acting Reversible Contraception [LARC]. https://www.colorado.gov/pacific/cdphe/cfpi-report. Accessed 6 July 2018.

Epstein, R. A. (1998). Chapter 1: Natural Law: The Utilitarian Connection. In *Principles for a free society: Reconciling individual liberty with the common good*. New York: Perseus Boos. https://archive.nytimes.com/www.nytimes.com/books/first/e/epstein-free.html. Accessed 6 July 2018.

Lepore, J. (2016). Baby Doe: A political history of tragedy. *The New Yorker*, February 1. https://www.newyorker.com/magazine/2016/02/01/baby-doe. Accessed 6 July 2018.

Chapter 14
What Should We Do?

Parenthood remains the greatest single preserve of the amateur.

Alvin Toffler, futurist

The family into which a child is born should not determine that child's opportunities in life.

John Rawls, political philosopher

Our society does not have a way of ensuring that genetic parents of children are competent and accountable, as we do for the parents of adopted children. Legal and physical custody of a newborn baby is given to anyone who conceived that child without regard for that person's ability to raise that child. We do not intervene until damage from abuse and/or neglect of that child comes to public attention even when we know that their newborn babies will enter the Cradle to Prison/Welfare-Dependency Pipeline so clearly described by the *Children's Defense Fund*. We support these parents and their children who later are incarcerated or are welfare dependent as adults. In Wisconsin, this accounts for 23% of state and 45% of county expenditures in addition to the resulting tragic lives (see Appendix 1).

Supporting vulnerable parents seems to be the most practical response to childbirth—but this does not change the following facts:

- Persons of any age who require custodians or guardians are not able to be responsible for their own lives.
- Adolescents are not adults and require legal and physical custodians—usually their parents.
- The 1st weeks, months, and years of life are critical in child development. Babies do not benefit from waiting for adolescent parents to mature.

We need to remind ourselves why the prevention of adolescent pregnancy is so important. Adolescent parenthood is an undesirable lifestyle in modern society. It is a cruel irony that while the American Humane Society restricts animal adoptions to adults, we accord parental rights to minors with the presumption that they are capable of entering parenthood on their own.

© Springer Nature Switzerland AG 2019

J. C. Westman, *Dealing with Child Abuse and Neglect as Public Health Problems*, https://doi.org/10.1007/978-3-030-05897-5_14

As a society, we actively try to prevent undesirable lifestyles. We devote public resources to preventing domestic violence, child neglect and abuse, drug abuse, alcoholism, smoking, obesity, sexually transmitted diseases, and adolescent pregnancy. When individuals persist in such behaviors despite interventions, we take one of two courses:

- When the resulting harm involves only the individual, we care for them. For example, our health-care systems help smokers and nonsmokers alike.
- When one's behavior harms others, such as with sexually transmitted diseases, our public health and law enforcement systems intervene. Adolescent parenthood has repercussions far beyond the adolescent parents. Its harmful effects— both short- and long-term—involve their babies, their families, and society.

Nonetheless, we automatically shift from adolescent pregnancy prevention to adolescent parent support based on our perceived lack of alternatives and our desire to minimize harm to the baby. Unfortunately, focusing only on the baby ignores the interests of the adolescent. Focusing only on the adolescent ignores the interests of the baby. In both situations, the interests of the larger family and society are ignored. Instead of these reactive, fragmented responses, the birth of babies to minors should first evoke consideration of the interests of the babies, then of the adolescents, then of their relatives, and ultimately of society.

Because our society holds no articulated expectations for parents who conceive and give birth to children, child neglect and abuse have reached epidemic proportions in the United States, exceeding that in all other developed nations. Enormous public expenditures on treatment, rehabilitation, and incarceration result. All of this would change dramatically if our vision for America was that all of our children will be raised by competent parents.

This vision could be achieved if we would value parenthood as a vital career that requires the basic managerial skills and resources essential for rearing children to become productive citizens. We could do this through instituting parenthood affirmation and certification as part of the Birth Certificate Application and as a tangible expression of a social contract between parents and society. This affirmation and contract that awards the legal and physical custody of a newborn could only be made by those who are not under the legal and physical custody of others. Wisconsin Cares, Inc., has proposed a feasible plan for implementing this explicit establishment of parental rights, which now are implicitly awarded to anyone who conceives a child without regard for that person's ability to assume the responsibilities in these rights (Wisconsin Cares 2016). This plan would interrupt the Cradle to Prison Pipeline.

We no longer can presume that everyone is capable of handling the responsibilities of parenthood until they damage a child through abuse and neglect. We no longer can regard a newborn baby as the personal property of the parents without the right as a US citizen to have an opportunity to succeed in life.

At some point in their lives, half of all children born in the United States will have lived in one-parent homes, mostly without fathers in their lives. Half of these children will live in poverty for a time and likely continue the cycle of family disadvantage. Without concerted action, every American taxpayer will continue to pay for the consequences. At this time, parents who raise a child to become a productive citizen contribute $1.4 million to our economy; parents who neglect and abuse a child who becomes a criminal or welfare dependent cost our economy $2.8 million (see Appendix 2).

Until we honor the right of all newborn babies to have an opportunity to succeed in life by having parents who are able to assume the responsibilities of raising them, our society will be burdened by the enormous human and financial costs of crime, violence, welfare dependency, and poverty. If we have the will and exercise common sense, we can shut off the Cradle to Prison/Welfare-Dependency Pipeline.

We no longer can afford to ignore the root causes of intergenerational poverty, crime, and welfare dependency in the United States. Based on the following facts, United Nations statistician Howard Friedman (212) carefully documented the declining international status of the United States in his book *The Measure of a Nation: How to Regain America's Competitive Edge and Boost Our Global Standing* (Friedman 2012):

- Americans have the lowest life expectancy among all comparable nations.
- Americans are at least two times more likely to be murdered and four times more likely to be incarcerated than any other comparable country.
- The United States shows the greatest disparity between rich and poor among all comparable nations.
- The United States is at the top of the list of comparable nations for child abuse and neglect rates and at the bottom for academic achievement.

While our nation focuses on current unemployment, the national debt and terrorism, the ailments that threaten the future of our society are being ignored. Especially dangerous is the decline in thriving families that will undermine the future prosperity and security of our nation. This decline in family well-being now deprives us of parents who can raise the next generation of productive citizens. At some point in their lives, half of all children born in the United States will have lived in one-parent homes, mostly without fathers. Half of these children will live in poverty for a time and may well continue the cycle of family disadvantage. Without concerted action, every American taxpayer will continue to pay for the consequences.

In sum, as it now stands:

- Parents who raise a child to become a productive citizen contribute $1.4 million to our economy; parents who neglect and abuse a child who becomes a criminal or welfare dependent cost our economy $2.8 million.
- Even though we know incompetent parents harm their babies, families, and society, we act as if we cannot intervene until their children have been damaged by abuse or neglect. Meanwhile, we continue to support these parents and their children at great cost with public and private funds.
- Adults who require custodians or guardians themselves because they are unable to care for themselves have full parental rights and the custody of their offspring.

- Adolescents who are not adults and require legal and physical custodians, usually their parents, have full parental rights and the custody of their offspring.
- The 1st weeks, months, and years of life are critical in child development. Babies simply cannot wait for dependent parents to mature or recover from disabilities if they are to have an opportunity to succeed in life.

We have not carefully thought through these issues. As a result, our responses are reactive rather than proactive. Child psychiatrist Paul Trad noted that adolescent childbirth is a "high-risk" crisis that warrants sensitive, realistic intervention (Trad 1993).

We need a paradigm that proactively protects the interests of everyone affected by adolescent childbirth. That paradigm is recognizing adolescent childbirth as a public health crisis. This principle also can be applied to childbirth by adults with legal guardians and adults adjudicated to be unfit parents. To counter advocates who regard intrusion on any parent's privacy as inappropriate paternalism, the idea of "soft paternalism" or "parentalism" has been advanced.

14.1 Soft Paternalism

Rebecca Maynard, professor of education and social policy at the University of Pennsylvania, suggests "soft paternalism" as the appropriate way to help people prone to self-defeating behaviors (Maynard n.d.). Missouri, for example, makes it illegal for persons identified as compulsive gamblers to enter casinos in order to help them break their addiction to gambling. Maynard suggests that "soft paternalism" be applied to adolescent pregnancy and childbirth as well.

Speed limits and traffic lights are two everyday examples of public interventions that protect us from the acts of others, as well as our own impulses. We likewise expect protection from unethical businesses and professionals. Only by restraining undesirable actions can we maintain a free society.

But paternalism, even soft paternalism, has a sexist flavor. It also evokes images of "big brother" or governmental control of private lives and even abuse of the disadvantaged. Such concerns become valid when a public policy has unintended consequences that override its benefits to society. This can happen with policies based on value judgments, such as "all cohabiting couples should be married."

However, this argument does not apply to policies based on scientific evidence, where demonstrated benefits unmistakably outweigh potential adverse effects. Such is the case with childbirth to adolescents and dependent adults. We need a less-controversial term that conveys the need to protect individuals through regulations that serve their interests.

I suggest the term parentalism. It conveys the need to protect and nurture. Our governments already apply parentalism in their *in loco parentis* role under the parens patriae doctrine. Specifically, it supports parental authority and limits the privileges of minors to prevent them from making irrevocable, life-altering decisions that they may later regret. Such interventions are needed when the stakes for society are high, as they are with adolescent and dependent adult childbirth.

We have precedents for establishing a legal relationship between a parent and a child in the application for a marriage license to the extent that marriage is seen as a precursor to parenthood. Most states have three requirements for establishing a legal marital relationship between two persons.

1. Affidavit: a declaration under oath that information provided is true and that no legal impediment exists to entering marriage:

   - Proof of age and residence eligibility
   - Information about previous marriages
   - Social Security number
   - Marriage is not between genetic relatives

2. License: authorizes the marriage ceremony after a waiting period.
3. Certificate of Marriage: executed by a legally authorized person.

Its vital importance to our society justifies setting similar minimum standards for the legal relationship between parent and child. This is critical now because of the incompetence of millions of contemporary parents. It is needed to align social values with integrative cultural values that further the common good through committed relationships between people.

Unlike the capacity to enter parenthood, legal marriage contracts are regulated at the state level. All except Mississippi set the age of consent at 18 without parental permission, but some states do allow for marriage with parental consent at younger ages. States tend to define the capacity to enter marriage as requiring less capacity than testamentary capacity or entering into a contract (Glezer and Devido 2017). Still, setting an age for marriage indirectly sets an age to enter parenthood, since childbirth usually accompanies marriage.

There has been much volatility in state drinking ages since the repeal of Prohibition in 1933. Shortly after the ratification of the 21st Amendment, which allowed individual states to regulate the commercial availability of alcoholic beverages, most states set their purchase ages at 21 since that was the voting age at the time. Most of these limits remained constant until the early 1970s. From 1969 to 1976, some 30 states lowered their purchase ages, generally to 18. This was primarily because the voting age was lowered from 21 to 18 in 1971 with the 12th Amendment. Twelve states kept their purchase ages at 21, set since the repeal of Prohibition, and never changed them. In 1984, Congress passed the National Minimum Drinking Age Act, which required states to raise their ages for purchase and public possession to 21 by October 1986 or lose 10% of their federal highway funds (Alcohol Policy Information System (APIS) n.d.).

The public currently supports parenthood through tax benefits, public education, and public assistance. To justify this support, we need greater parental accountability. We should link the public benefits of parenthood to a person's capacity to fulfill its responsibilities.

The capacity to conceive and give birth says nothing about a parent's competence to rear a child. We need to determine a parent's capability to handle the responsibilities of parenthood by setting a minimum standard based on our cultural expectations of parenthood.

Setting a standard for parenthood is justified on two grounds: a police power to maintain political stability and order and a parens patriae power to protect the welfare of those unable to act in their own best interests, such as minors or the mentally incompetent.

James Dwyer, professor of law at William and Mary University, proposes that certain categories of high-risk parents be required to apply for certification that they meet a minimum standard to become the legal and physical custodians of their children (Dwyer 2009; Roberts 1996). This minimum standard would stem from the principle that a person who requires a legal and physical custodian or guardian or who is legally unfit to parent cannot be the legal and physical custodian of a child. Dwyer points out that newborn babies have a moral right and a constitutional right under the Due Process Clause of the Fourteenth Amendment against the state placing them into a legal relationship with birth parents known to be unfit.

Most commonly, this would involve those who require legal and physical custodians because they are legal minors. Less commonly, it also would include those with developmental disabilities or mental illnesses and those who are incarcerated for violent crimes or adjudicated to be unfit parents.

Legal standards for decision-making competence, custodianship, and guardianship vary across jurisdictions. Generally, they embody the ability to understand relevant information and consequences, to make choices through mature reasoning, and to communicate these choices. The criteria for obtaining a marriage license address these capacities. Mental health professionals use additional tools for assessing the competency of mentally ill and developmentally disabled parents.

A Birth Certificate is a vital record akin to a Marriage Certificate. Issued shortly after birth, it usually results when the mother's health-care provider files the required forms with a state agency. It contains detailed information about the birth, baby, parents, and family histories. It could also signify that the parents are committed to parenthood and meet minimum standards for legal and physical custodianship of the newborn. The Birth Certificate process could be modified to affirm that our society places a high enough value on parenthood to certify that every newborn has a parent who meets minimum standards for parenthood.

Following Dwyer's reasoning, potential high-risk parents would be identified as soon as possible before childbirth. This could be done by combining the health, child welfare, and correctional and birth registration systems to make the Birth Certificate process meaningful for the well-being of the newborn. This process could be initiated at one of three points. In order of desirability, they are:

1. When pregnancy is diagnosed
2. When prenatal care begins
3. On admission to a hospital or birthing center

At the first point of contact, professionals could note the age of the mother and check databases for child abuse and neglect and relevant correctional records. Even in the event the pregnancy is terminated, this would ensure that the pregnancy becomes part of state and national health statistics. Indeed, some states already require reporting of pregnancy terminations and fetal deaths.

The Birth Certificate could be modified to become a certificate of parenthood conveying legal and physical custodianship. Because the babies of minor parents do not have legal and physical custodians, this would involve creating a statutory requirement that babies born before the mother attains a certain age, such as 17 1/2, be assigned legal and physical custodians.

In 1988, the Institute of Medicine defined public health as what we, as a society, do collectively to assure the conditions for people to be healthy (IOM 1988; Mailman School of Public Health n.d.). Wisconsin Cares, Inc., an advocacy organization for children and families, proposes that the public health primary, secondary, and tertiary prevention practice models be applied to child abuse and neglect in order to prevent the formation of the Cradle to Prison/Welfare-Dependency Pipeline and resulting intergenerational poverty (Wisconsin Cares 2016).

Primary prevention means preventing child abuse and neglect in the first place as with immunization for diseases. Secondary prevention means treating child abuse and neglect. Tertiary prevention means reducing damage that has occurred. This can be done by setting a simple, clear-cut standard for awarding the legal and physical custody of a newborn baby, who is a person with a right to have an opportunity to become a productive citizen as advocated by the US Declaration of Independence and Constitution. This standard simply would be that the parent not be under the legal physical custody or guardianship of another person and, therefore, be competent to manage her or his own life before assuming responsibility for the life of a newborn baby.

14.2   Primary Prevention

Current law assumes that all parents, regardless of age or other dependency, are the legal and physical custodians of their children unless a court determines otherwise. However, by definition minor parents are dependent persons who require their own legal and physical custodians. While they cannot legally be responsible for their own lives, they now are regarded as the legal and physical custodians of their newborn babies unless a court awards custody to another person(s). As a result, grandparents often care for grandchildren without legal authority to make medical and other important decisions for the children. Wisconsin Statute §49.90 (called the grandparent liability law) provides that a parent has an obligation to maintain or support the child of a dependent person under the age of 18 even though they do not have custody of that child (Wisconsin Statutes 2018). Similarly, adults with guardians and adults who are under the legal and physical custody of the state are the legal and physical custodians of their newborn child unless a court determines otherwise.

Especially problematic are women who give birth while incarcerated. In each of these instances, unnecessary burdens are created for child protection agencies and courts. In addition, all states presume that parents are responsible for the well-being of their children but do not require informing parents of their responsibilities, except in divorce or other child custody actions.

The objective of primary prevention is that every child will have a parent as legal and physical custodian who understands and accepts and can carry out the responsibilities of parenthood. To that end, we would:

- Apply the public health principle of primary prevention to social problems by preventing the formation of vulnerable families.
- Shift the focus from remediation to prevention.
- Stimulate thinking about the rights of newborn babies.
- Develop a process for the affirmation of parenthood responsibilities.

These objectives would be met by ensuring that:

- Every newborn baby's parent/custodian is fully aware of the responsibilities of parenthood and the consequences of failing to meet them.
- Whenever parents are in the custody of other persons, such as a minor or an incarcerated or legally incompetent adult, that fact creates a presumption that these parents cannot be the legal and physical custodians of their newborn babies.
- Parenthood Planning Counseling is provided for dependent parents and their families when the decision is made to continue the dependent person's pregnancy to childbirth.
- When a parent is not legally competent for any reason, a qualified custodian, such as the parent of the dependent parent (the grandparent of the newborn), if willing and able, is permitted to assume legal custody of the newborn baby.

14.3   Parenthood Affirmation

The Birth Certificate Application would include a paragraph setting forth the minimum standards for parenthood commonly used by family courts, which are basically to:

- Provide sufficient income independently or with public assistance for the child's clothing, shelter, education, health care, social, and recreational activities.
- Provide the love, security, and emotional support necessary for the healthy development of the child.
- Foster the child's intellectual, social, and moral development.
- Socialize the child by setting limits and encouraging civil behavior and by protecting the child from physical, emotional, and social harm.

The inclusion of these responsibilities in the Birth Certificate Application would offer an opportunity for all parents to affirm their awareness of the responsibilities of parenthood, to evaluate their capacities to meet them, and to obtain information about available parenting resources. The existing Birth Certificate Application process would be advanced in time to begin when a pregnancy is diagnosed and the decision is made to continue it to childbirth in order to insure:

1. That the birth mother and father of a child are legally competent to manage her or his own affairs (i.e., is not under the legal and physical custody or guardianship of another—usually that person's parent or the state). This presumption may be rebutted by a termination of parental rights (TPR) action or any other legal determination of unfitness of a mother or father.

2. Whenever any pregnant person chooses to continue her pregnancy to childbirth, she and the father, if known, would be informed of the responsibilities of parenthood as outlined in the Birth Certificate Application and asked to acknowledge awareness and understanding of those responsibilities by signing the following Parenthood Affirmation:

   I am aware of, understand and accept the responsibilities of parenthood. _____ (name of parent) _____ (co-signer when applicable)

   A person who requires a legal and physical custodian or guardian or who has been adjudicated to be legally unfit to assume the responsibilities of parenthood would not be qualified to sign this affirmation alone and would require a qualified cosigner. (Nonmarital fathers may now voluntarily, or be required to legally, acknowledge their financial support obligations. That acknowledgment would include an awareness of their other parental responsibilities as well.) By signing awareness of the responsibilities of parenthood, a qualified person would be presumed to be accepting the responsibilities of parenthood as the legal and physical custodian of the newborn baby. If qualified persons decline to sign that section of the Birth Certificate Application, the person administering the form would note on the application that those parents had been informed of their responsibilities and had declined to sign the application. This would trigger the mandatory reporting of a child suspected to be in need of protective services. For example, in Wisconsin this is required by State Statute 48.13.

3. At the time dependent persons' pregnancies are diagnosed and the decision is made to continue to childbirth, Parenthood Planning Counseling would be required for the dependent persons and their families. Such counseling can be activated by family planning and prenatal services that have access to pregnant adolescents and dependent adults. A mandated reporting process would be triggered as soon as an adolescent or dependent adult learns of her pregnancy and decides to continue to childbirth. This process would have three potential outcomes:

   - The custodians or guardians of the dependent parents would cosign the Parenthood Affirmation and continue the custody of the dependent parents and assume the custody of the newborn babies if they are willing and able to do so and meet the standards of Kinship Care (Glezer and Devido 2017). The qualified custodian(s) or guardian(s) would be the legal and physical custodian(s) of the newborn child until the mother or father attains legal age or a dependent adult becomes self-sufficient.

- The dependent parents and their families would make a voluntary adoption plan effective at birth.
- If at the time the pregnancy is diagnosed, it is evident there is no qualified person(s) who is willing and able to assume the newborn's custody, the unborn child will be presumed to be without a custodial parent at birth. A Child in Need of Protection action would then take the necessary steps for the state to assume legal and physical custody of the newborn child, and an adoption plan would be made effective at the birth of the baby.

14.4 Parenthood Certification

In the proposed certification process, when a pregnancy is identified and the decision is made to continue to childbirth, those eligible for automatic certification would be informed about making a Parenthood Affirmation. Those ineligible for automatic certification would be contacted by a child welfare worker. A Parenthood Planning Team would be formed to counsel them and their families.

Wisconsin Cares, Inc., proposes that Parenthood Certification be implemented by modifying the Birth Certificate so that it also becomes a Parenthood Certificate that formally affirms legal and physical custodianship of the child (Glezer and Devido 2017).

This model would be implemented by identifying dependent mothers and fathers at the earliest possible time. The birth registration process would be expanded to include affirmation that a parent has made a commitment to carry out the responsibilities of parenthood. This would include:

1. Automatic certification of parenthood for mothers and fathers who are adults and sign the Parenthood Affirmation
2. A certification application and review process when a mother or father is:

   (a) A legal minor under 17 ½ at due date
   (b) Developmentally disabled or mentally ill adult with a guardian
   (c) Adjudicated as an unfit parent because of child neglect or abuse
   (d) Currently incarcerated

Adults who require custodians or guardians and minors who require legal and physical custodians, usually their parents, because they are unable to care for themselves, would be presumed in a state's Children's Code to be ineligible to assume the legal and physical custody of a newborn baby with attendant parental rights.

The first professional who becomes aware of a dependent person's decision to continue a pregnancy would contact the child welfare system. A Parenthood Planning Team would be formed and activate the Parenthood Certification process through Parenthood Planning Counseling. Federal law already requires in-hospital paternity acknowledgment programs to establish a baby's paternity at birth.

For the dependent parent, Parenthood Planning Counseling would include identifying adults qualified to assume legal and physical custodianship of the newborn baby or making an adoption plan. The team would help adults interested in custodianship determine if they are capable of assuming the following custodianship responsibilities:

1. Continue to provide legal and physical custodianship of the dependent mother or father.
2. Provide childrearing resources, including shelter, clothing, and food for the mother or father and baby.
3. Advocate for the parent and the baby, including the ability to provide health care.

If they are willing and able to do so, they would be the legal and physical custodians recorded on the Birth Certificate by cosigning the Parenthood Affirmation.

When no adult family member is willing and able to assume legal and physical custodianship of the newborn child, a Child in Need of Protection Services petition would be filed. A court would appoint a guardian ad litem to the Parenthood Planning Team. The guardian ad litem would represent the unborn baby, seek termination of parental rights, and make an adoption plan. The Birth Certificate would record a state or private agency as the legal and physical custodian until the adoption is finalized.

If an adolescent or dependent adult gives birth without prenatal care, the hospital now can immediately refer the case to child welfare services. The lack of prenatal care itself constitutes medical neglect that requires investigation and is grounds for automatic termination of parental rights followed by adoption. The state is recorded

Table 14.1 Model for a parenthood certification process

Model for a parenthood certification process	
Automatic certification	Certification of cosigner by application
Adults	1. Minors with or without parents (legal and physical custodians)
	2. Adults with guardians
	3. Adults adjudicated as unfit parents
	4. Adults current incarcerated
Procedure	Procedure
Sign Parenthood Pledge with birth registration application	1. Parenthood planning team is formed to provide parenthood planning counseling at the time pregnancy is diagnosed
	2. Formulation of a voluntary adoption plan is considered
	3. Qualified relative is cosigner of the parenthood pledge and becomes the temporary or permanent legal and physical custodian of the newborn baby
	4. If there is no relative qualified to be a legal and physical custodian, a guardian ad litem is appointed to institute an involuntary termination of parental rights with an adoption plan at birth

as the legal and physical custodian until an individual is appointed as custodian or the adoption is finalized (Table 14.1).

The goal is to act before birth in determining who will have the legal and physical custody of a newborn baby when there are questions about a parent's capacity to assume that responsibility.

We no longer can presume that everyone is capable of handling the responsibilities of parenthood until they damage a child through abuse and neglect. We no longer can regard a newborn baby as the personal property of the parents without the right as a US citizen to have an opportunity to succeed in life.

Until we honor the right of all newborn babies to have an opportunity to succeed in life by having parents who are able to assume the responsibilities of raising them, our society will be burdened by the enormous human and financial costs of crime, violence, welfare dependency, and poverty. If we have the will and exercise common sense, we can shut off the Cradle to Prison/Welfare-Dependency Pipeline.

14.5   Objections to a Certification Process

This proposal will face resistance because it appears to add new burdens to legal and social service systems already strained by responding to child neglect and abuse. It invokes images of government restrictions of individual liberties, the invasion of family privacy, and the stigmatization of dependent parents. Some adults might feel insulted by being required to sign the Parenthood Affirmation even though they would not feel that way about any other licensing or contract process.

Allegations of "genocide" of minorities and punishing people living in poverty also can be expected. It might even appear to presume guilt unless innocence is proved for those believe that the role of government is limited to intervening after harms have occurred. It might place health-care professionals in the position of reporting pregnancies and conflict with their ethical codes.

None of these objections are substantive or valid. Establishing eligibility to make the Parenthood Pledge is not:

1. *Eugenics*: It does not affect conception except as it causes people to think more seriously about conceiving and raising a child.
2. *Against the human right to procreate*: The survival of the species mandates the right of every human being to procreate, but the survival of the species also depends upon the ability of a parent to fulfill the duty to competently raise a child that is inherent in that right.
3. *Racist*: Weighting toward minority groups is coincidental, not targeted. Most minority parents are competent parents.
4. *Discrimination against the poor*: Weighting toward the disadvantaged is coincidental. Many parents living in poverty are competent parents.
5. *Elitist*: Wealthy parents can be incompetent.

6. *An unconstitutional invasion of the privacy of the family*: There is no Constitutional basis for parental rights other than as inferred from the Fourth Amendment's protection of the privacy of the home and the Fourteen Amendment's due process clause. In fact, there is a Constitutional basis for children's right to have an opportunity to succeed in life. Parenthood Certification would explicitly and officially affirm parental rights with attendant responsibilities in the Birth Certificate. Parenthood Affirmation would explicitly award now implicit parental rights and call attention to their accompanying responsibilities. States now have the power to set and regulate family policies as expressed in child abuse and neglect, child custody, and termination of parental rights statutes.

7. An *intrusion on individual liberty*: States have the responsibility to regulate individual actions that can potentially harm other persons through establishing qualifications and licensing, such as through licensing motor vehicle drivers, trades, and professions. Parents are not at liberty to harm their children.

8. *Impractical*: Parenthood Affirmation can be easily incorporated in the birth registration application and become a certification of parenthood in the Birth Certificate.

9. *Costly*: The volume of Parenthood Planning Counseling would increase the number of professionals needed to implement it. However, the immediate savings in health-care costs and the short- and long-term savings in educational, mental health, social services, and correctional costs would far offset those comparatively infinitesimal costs.

Certifying a person's qualification for parenthood would demonstrate that our society places a high value on ensuring that all children have competent parents. It would signal that we recognize parenthood as a valued and vital career for which we have established a minimum standard.

14.6   A Feasible Plan

Since adolescents gradually assume adult responsibilities, we set ages for awarding each responsibility. Because of the impact adolescent childbirth has on our society and because the average age of menarche is 12, we must establish an age at which parenthood can be entered and the legal and physical custodianship of a newborn baby can be assumed. This is particularly important because adolescent parenthood raises a baby's risk of prematurity, morbidity, developmental problems, and neglect and/or abuse. The most sensible and realistic approach is to recognize dependent-parent childbirth as the serious public health crisis that it is.

In our culture, dependent parenthood is undesirable for parents and babies. In spite of this, we provide financial, educational, and group home support for adolescent mothers and their babies who too often are harmed despite the support.

The most striking aspect of adolescent and dependent adult childbirth is that the newborn baby does not have a qualified legal and physical custodian.

Without creating a new bureaucracy, we can organize Parenthood Planning Teams from family planning, prenatal care, child welfare, home visitation, and legal programs that already exist. We can follow the model of crisis intervention teams that address other health and child welfare matters. Parenthood Planning Teams can guide adolescents and dependent adults and their families to make sound decisions as is already required for federal Adolescent Family Life Demonstration Projects.

The goal is to act before birth. When a dependent parent's baby is born, three reasonable outcomes exist:

1. Relatives continue custodianship of the dependent parent and assume temporary or permanent custodianship of the newborn baby.
2. The dependent parents and their families make a voluntary adoption plan.
3. A Parenthood Planning Team makes an involuntary adoption plan for the baby when relatives are unwilling and/or unable to assume custodianship of the dependent mother and her baby. Adoption offers the most practical and available access to competent parents for babies who do not have competent parents.

Most importantly, the Parenthood Pledge and Parenthood Certification would be concrete symbols of our society's devotion to our children and to our own future prosperity. In addition to the long-term result of providing an opportunity for success in life for newborn babies, it would have the short-term effect of removing the status and financial and other supportive benefits that provide incentives for dependent persons to give birth and to become parents.

14.7   Strengthening Communities

In his book *Uneasy Peace: The Great Crime Decline, the Renewal of City Life, and the Next War on Violence*, Patrick Sharkey offers the cheering possibility of spending money to rebuild communities and replacing the noxious "warrior cop" with "community building quarterbacks" (Sharkey 2018).

Single motherhood is one of four risks for poverty, which includes unemployment, low levels of education, and forming households at young ages (Brady et al. 2018). In the majority of comparable nations, single mothers are not more likely to be poor. Denmark, for example, has chosen to provide universal cash benefits and tax credits for children, publicly subsidized child care and health care, and paid parental leave. Because of these generous social policies, single mothers and their children have a level of economic security similar to that of other families.

14.8 Secondary Prevention

The AVANCE program offers parents a continuum of services beginning with the Parent-Child Education Program (PCEP) as the point of entry. Progression through PCEP is an educational and growth program for parents and children through community collaborations and partnerships. After graduation, AVANCE helps parents enroll in GED, ESL, college courses, and job training and certification programs.

Early Childhood Family Education (ECFE) is a program for all Minnesota families with children from birth to kindergarten with entrance offered through Minnesota public school districts (Minnesota Department of Education n.d.). ECFE recognizes that the family provides a child's first and most significant learning environment and that parents are a child's first and most important teachers. ECFE's goal is to enhance the ability of all parents and other family members to provide the best possible environment for their children's learning and growth.

The Help Me Grow system is designed to help states and communities leverage resources to insure that they identify vulnerable children, link families to community-based services, and empower families to support their children's healthy development through the implementation of four Core Components: (1) child health-care provider outreach, (2) family and community outreach, (3) centralized access point, and (4) ongoing data collection and analysis (Help Me Grow 2018).

Prevent Child Abuse Tennessee offers home-based programs to vulnerable families, crisis intervention, parent-to-parent empowerment, and public education about prevention (PCAT, n.d.). Each program aims to reduce traumatic experiences resulting from unsafe adult behavior and environments that can weaken any child's foundation. Preventing abuse and neglect from happening in the first place gives children the best chance at successful futures.

14.9 Conclusion

Setting a minimum standard for parenthood and certifying that it has been met would indicate that our society places a high value on protecting its Posterity and economic prosperity by ensuring that all children have parents who can raise them to become productive citizens. It would signal that we recognize parenthood as a valued career for which we have established a minimum standard. It would help to ensure that every newborn has an opportunity to become a productive citizen. It would reduce early childhood adversity and curtail the Cradle to Prison Pipeline.

Without creating a new bureaucracy, we can provide Parenthood Planning Counseling for pregnant dependent persons and their families through family planning, prenatal care, child welfare, home visitation, and coordinated services/ Wraparound programs that already exist. We can follow the counseling model already required for federal Adolescent Family Life Demonstration Projects. Only through ensuring that all newborn babies have parents who are capable of raising them can we fulfill the Parenthood-Society Contract and ensure the future prosperity of our nation.

We know that adolescents gradually learn to assume adult responsibilities, and so, we set ages for awarding these responsibilities. Because of the great impact that adolescent childbirth has on our society and because the average age of the onset of menarche now is 12, we must establish an age at which legal and physical custodianship (parenthood) for a child can be acquired.

In our modern society, dependent parenthood is an undesirable lifestyle for both parents and babies. In spite of this, we provide financial, educational, and group home support for adolescent mothers in an effort to help them function as parents. We do this with the intent of helping their babies, who still are harmed in spite of the support provided.

The most striking aspect of adolescent and dependent adult childbirth is that the newborn baby does not have a qualified legal and physical custodian. This is particularly significant because adolescent parenthood clearly raises a baby's risk of prematurity, morbidity, developmental problems, neglect, and abuse.

The most sensible and realistic approach is to recognize dependent-parent childbirth as the serious public health crisis it is. Without creating a new bureaucracy, we can organize Parenthood Planning Teams composed of professionals in the existing fields of family planning, prenatal care, child welfare, home visitation, and law. We can do so following the model of the crisis intervention teams that currently address other health and child welfare matters. These Parenthood Planning Teams can guide adolescents and dependent adults and their families in making the most appropriate decisions for all concerned. The goal is to act before birth to avoid the adverse conditions that would otherwise harm the newborn baby.

When a dependent parent's baby is born, there are three reasonable outcomes after all those involved have carefully considered the options and consequences: (1) relatives continue legal and physical custodianship of the dependent mother and assume temporary legal and physical custodianship of the baby, (2) the dependent parents and their families make a voluntary adoption plan for the baby, or (3) a Parenthood Planning Team makes an involuntary adoption plan for the baby when relatives cannot assume legal and physical custodianship of the dependent mother and her baby. Adoption offers the most practical and available access to competent parents for babies who do not have competent parents.

Setting minimum standards for parenthood by modifying Birth Certification to become a Parenthood Certification process as well would signify that our society places a high value on ensuring that all of our children have competent parents and thereby ensuring the prosperity of our nation.

References

Alcohol Policy Information System (APIS), National Institute on Alcohol Abuse and Alcoholism (NIAAA). (n.d.). The 1984 national minimum drinking age act. https://alcoholpolicy.niaaa.nih.gov/the-1984-national-minimum-drinking-age-act. Accessed 19 Oct 2018.

Brady, D., Finnigan, R. M., & Hubgen, S. (2018, February 11). Single mothers are not the problem. *The New York Times Sunday Review*.

Dwyer, J. G. (2009). Constitutional birthright: The state, parentage, and the rights of newborn persons. *Faculty Publications*. 26. http://scholarship.law.wm.edu/facpubs/26/. Accessed 6 July 2018.

Friedman, H. S. (2012). *The measure of a nation: How to regain America's competitive edge and boost our global standing*. Amherst: Prometheus Books.

Glezer, A., & Devido, J. J. (2017). Evaluation of the capacity to marry. *The Journal of the American Academy of Psychiatry and the Law, 45*, 292–297. http://jaapl.org/content/45/3/292. Accessed 6 July 2018.

Help Me Grow National Center, Connecticut Children's Medical Center. The HUG System Model. (2018). https://helpmegrownational.org/what-is-help-me-grow/hmg-system-model/. Accessed 6 July 2018.

IOM [Institute of Medicine]. (1988). *The future of public health*. Washington, DC: National Academies Press. https://www.nap.edu/catalog/1091/the-future-of-public-health. Accessed 6 July 2018.

Mailman School of Public Health, Columbia University. (n.d.). What is public health? https://www.mailman.columbia.edu/public-health-now/news/what-public-health-introduction. Accessed 6 July 2018.

Maynard, R. (n.d.). *Three P: Paternalism, teenage pregnancy prevention, and teenage parent services*. University of Maryland School of Public Policy Welfare Reform Academy. http://www.welfareacademy.org/conf/papers/maynard_.shtml. Accessed 6 July 2018.

Minnesota Department of Education. (n.d.). Early childhood family education. https://education.mn.gov/MDE/fam/elsprog/ECFE/. Accessed 6 July 2018.

PCAT [Prevent Child Abuse Tennessee] (n.d.). http://www.pcat.org/. Accessed 6 July 2018.

Roberts, M. A. (1996). Parent and child in conflict: Between liberty and responsibility. *Notre Dame Journal of Ethics & Public Policy, 10*(2), 485. http://scholarship.law.nd.edu/ndjlepp/vol10/iss2/2. Accessed 6 July 2018.

Sharkey, P. (2018). *Uneasy peace: The great crime decline, the renewal of city life, and the next war on violence*. New York: Norton.

Trad, P. (1993). Adolescent pregnancy: An intervention challenge. *Child Psychiatry and Human Development, 24*(2), 99–113.

Wisconsin Cares, Inc. (2016). Protecting our most precious asset: our youngest citizens. A place to start: The affirmation of parenthood. http://www.wisconsincares.net/wp-content/uploads/2016/03/Parenthood_Affirmation_Proposal_11-15.pdf. Accessed 6 July 2018.

Wisconsin Statutes. (2018). 49.90 liability of relatives; enforcement. https://docs.legis.wisconsin.gov/statutes/statutes/49/VI/90. Accessed 6 July 2018.

Chapter 15
Barriers to Change and Hope for the Future

When reality is unpleasant, illusions offer an attractive escape route. In difficult times unscrupulous manipulators enjoy a competitive advantage over those who seek to confront reality.

George Soros (2011)

The most important barriers to constructive social change are (1) "totalism," (2) reactions to instability and human differences, (3) the financial benefits of status quo inefficiency, (4) weak social capital, (5) the failure of families and schools to develop the analytic and collaborative skills individuals need for teamwork, and (6) mistrust of government institutions.

15.1 Totalism

The greatest barrier to constructive social change is what Psychohistorian Robert Jay Lifton called totalism (Lifton 1989). This occurs when political or religious systems seek to stamp out independent thought. Totalism is particularly attractive when systems are on the edge of chaos. When we are confronted by something so big it requires us to change the way we think and the way we see the world, denial is a natural response. Denial keeps our minds from becoming overloaded.

An example of totalism is the polarization of political parties. At a time when the public is open to changes, both political parties have become more rigid by representing special interest groups that trump the common good by encouraging opposition to, rather than interaction with, people with different ideas. This promotes single-mindedness and resistance to problem-solving, which involves collaboration and teamwork.

© Springer Nature Switzerland AG 2019
J. C. Westman, *Dealing with Child Abuse and Neglect as Public Health Problems*, https://doi.org/10.1007/978-3-030-05897-5_15

15.2   Instability and Human Differences

As psychiatrist Denis Donovan pointed out to me, if there's anything Americans can't stand, it's instability. Just when a system, such as education, mental health, health care, or human services, is loosening up enough to reorganize itself, it destabilizes. We jump in to stabilize the system and prevent adaptive reorganization. When that system fails to reorganize, it then is seen as seriously flawed and becomes more unstable.

At the level of individual differences, Princeton Social Psychologist Susan Fiske says that two emotions lie at the heart of a vast number of interpersonal, societal, and international tensions: envy and scorn (Price 2010). Our human tendency is to compare ourselves to others and to compare our group to other groups. We envy people who are higher in competence and/or power. We scorn people who are lower in competence and/or power either by pitying or being disgusted with them.

In groups, these emotions spawn stereotypes that lead to prejudice and discrimination…especially during stressful times. Globally, the United States is widely perceived as powerful and thus can face envy and distrust from other parts of the world. Within the United States, educated people can be scorned as impractical or out of touch. Uneducated persons can be seen as lacking intelligence.

Gender differences are particularly relevant when it comes to childbirth and childrearing. Women can see men as being biased and vice versa. Homemaking roles are especially associated with male and female stereotypes. The fact that males simply conceive and females conceive and bear children has powerful effects on the way that people perceive motherhood and fatherhood. This spills over into negative reactions of females to proposals made by males and vice versa.

15.3   The Financial Benefits of Inefficiency

In 1961, President Dwight Eisenhower warned about the military-industrial complex that spawned unnecessary projects and costs. In 1965, Secretary of Defense Robert McNamara highlighted how the efficiency of a system, in this case the military forces, was less important than expansion of private sector defense expenditures (McNamara and Van De Mark 1996). A similar case can be made for service industries that depend upon the products of incompetent parents.

Today our nation is shining a bright light on the economics of the conflict between cutting public costs and creating and saving jobs. For example, most of the money related to the "get tough on crime" movement is spent on imprisonment which creates jobs. This means cutting funds for prevention, treatment, education, and resources that would keep over half the prisoners with mental illnesses and drug problems out of prison in the first place. Efforts are made to keep prisons open even when they no longer are needed to maintain local jobs and businesses. Job security trumps cutting incarceration costs. A hidden agenda of get-tough-on-crime policies can even be to imprison as many people as possible to support local economies and to privatize public prisons.

Moreover, the health care, mental health, and human services systems are highly fragmented. This leads to redundancy, inefficiency, and reduced efficacy. Primary health-care and mental health clinicians have been locked into traditions that separate them. About 65% of Americans are overweight or obese, and most are resistant to weight loss. The excess weight costs our nation an estimated $93 billion in medical bills every year. If these systems functioned more efficiently and focused on prevention, overall costs would be reduced significantly. But this also means that anyone who would lose revenue has an incentive to ignore reforming these systems.

Today, psychiatry and psychology are not calling for social policies and neighborhood interventions that shield children from stressors that weaken families and limit the growth, health, learning, and wellbeing of entire populations. Instead the focus is on brain development, the early diagnosis of problems and medications.

Finally, collaboration inside bureaucracies is a concept more often lauded than enacted. Rigid funding pathways (silos), tradition, and territoriality stand in the way. Even communities with a long history of activism struggle with getting groups that can learn from each other to plan projects for their mutual benefit. At the same time, in her book *Quiet*, Susan Cain (2012) points out that efforts to force collaboration through offices without walls, structured groupthink, and confusing social skills with the ability to work in teams can backfire when constant interruptions kill creativity.

Here is a typical example of collaborative failure at the state level from my personal experience. In April 2000, Wisconsin Governor Tommy Thompson created the Governor's Blue-Ribbon Commission on State-Local Partnerships for the twenty-first century. He charged it with conducting a "mini-constitutional convention" to rethink what Wisconsin government does and how it can perform better with less money. In January of 2001, the Commission laid out a bold strategy that emphasized innovative partnerships among Wisconsin's state and local governments. The strategy aimed to improve the quality of life for all state citizens and deliver better value for taxpayers' dollars. It would have reduced tension in the political system and made Wisconsin's state and local governments genuine partners instead of adversaries. Over the following decade, few of its proposals saw the light of day.

15.4 Weak Social Capital

Weakened social capital is seen in things that have vanished almost unnoticed from our society…neighborhood parties and get-togethers with friends, the unconditional kindness of strangers, and a shared pursuit of the public good rather than the solitary quest for private goods.

Harvard Professor of Public Policy Robert Putnam (2001) noted in his book *Bowling Alone* that the changing character of work and the closely related flow of women into the workforce were among the most far-reaching upheavals of the twentieth century (Putnam 2001). This workplace transformation was comparable to the metamorphosis of America from a nation of farms to one of factories and offices. Public and private American institutions and norms as well as workplace practices have only begun to adapt to the shift of mothers from homes to workplaces. This workplace revolution contributed to the decline in face-to-face social connectedness and civic involvement now aggravated by communication through social media. At the same time, the social media do offer the potential for changing perceptions and stimulating constructive actions.

15.5   Lack of Analytic and Collaborative Skills

David Boulton, learning technologist and creator of Children of the Code, asks how families, schools, and social support systems might differ if their central organizing principle was driven by how well children learn to solve problems rather than how well they learn outdated, adult-centric lessons (Children of the Code 2018).

Even intelligent and well-educated people accept information from an apparently authoritative source rather than thinking analytically. If a statement begins, "Neuroscience tells us that" then finishes with nonsense, a significant percentage will simply accept it. If the same assertion is made without reference to neuroscience, they recognize that the statement makes no sense. Our perceptions of reality are dependent upon the beliefs we hold. This is belief-dependent "reality."

At a more personal level, Boulton points out that most children who struggle with learning to read English believe *something is wrong with themselves ... something to be ashamed of. Unintentionally but pervasively, parents, schools, and society contribute to this myth*. Children do not think that the trouble might be normal differences in their *genes and brains* in the same way people can be tall or short. They do not suspect that their *parents, siblings, and caregivers might not have engaged them enough in conversation* before they started school. They do not wonder if their teachers did not teach them well. They do not know that the complicated English language presents an unnatural processing challenge. *They blame themselves. They feel ashamed of themselves*...ashamed of their minds. Statements like "I'm dumb," "I'm stupid," and "I'm not good in school" reflect their shame.

Walking, talking, reading, writing, math, science, art, politics, philosophy, physical health, emotional wellbeing, financial security, upward mobility, family harmony, social responsibility, and spiritual attunement ... there is not any human activity that is not enhanced and constrained by learning. Learning how to think critically and to solve problems is as relevant to personal, corporate, national, and world problem-solving as it is to a parent's love, achieving an individual's potential and the quest for scientific, artistic, philosophical, and spiritual truths. The most practical and profound response to ambiguities in school, at home, on the job, and in society is to learn how to invent and reinvent ... the foundation of collaboration and teamwork.

Today's young people generally have had more structure than any other generation in American history. They are supervised, coached, and tutored to prepare them for success in school. Students are encouraged to follow personal passions and dreams to align themselves with American individualism.

Most contemporary young adults will not get married, buy a house, and have children in the sequence followed by previous generations. Most will spend a decade searching for their roles in our society. Many are unprepared for an uncertain, open world in which success is determined by their usefulness to others.

In order to succeed, they will discover that the purpose of their life is not to find themselves by pursuing their passions. Instead, it is to lose themselves in serving others. The flourishing young adult commits to a spouse and a community. Genuine success in life is not achieved from satisfying our inner world desires but from our significance to others in our outer world.

15.6   Mistrust of Government Institutions

There are good reasons for concern about government overreaching in family and juvenile behavioral matters. Examples range from the notorious misuse and failures of foster care to overreaction to the 2012 Newton, Connecticut, school shooting though "zero tolerance" of such behavior as pointing a finger and pretending to shoot a classmate.

As this book has demonstrated, the failure of government institutions to intervene in family lives in a timely and appropriate manner is a far greater concern than governmental overreaching. Still, no public or private system operates perfectly. For this reason, involuntary actions arising from Parenthood Planning Counseling and Parenthood Affirmation are designed to include the checks and balances of the courts, such as by appointing a guardian ad litem for the unborn child when an involuntary adoption is planned at birth.

15.7   The Good News

In his book *The Evolution of Virtue, Altruism, and Shame*, Christopher Boehm (2012) presents evidence for the evolution of the human capacity for bonding, collaboration, and altruism. As collaboration was necessary for efficient hunting, natural selection favored individuals who were better at inhibiting their own antisocial tendencies, either through fear of punishment or through absorbing and identifying with their group's rules. Competition, territoriality, and tribalism rooted in our reptilian brains served humans well in less complicated worlds but so did cooperation and the ability to trust and bond rooted in our forebrains. While competition is a key driver in human evolution and human affairs, collaboration and teamwork are equally if not more important.

In her book *Building a Win-Win World*, economist Hazel Henderson (1996) offers hope for the future global economy. She demonstrates how the present global economy is unsustainable because of its negative effects on employees, families, communities, and our ecosystem. She sees a shift taking place from a value system based on competition, conflict, and what she calls "economism" (an approach that puts economics at the center of public policy and reduces individual and public choices to matters of self-interest and profit) toward a value system based on interdependence, sustainability, and cooperation. In her view, a "quality-of-life" language is emerging that opens the way for new approaches to our national and global problems. There is "slow-motion good news" going on, she says, as the old ways of doing things are challenged by "global citizens," grassroots organizations, and enlightened businesses around the world.

15.8 Human Natural Capital

Our focus on enhancing our nonhuman natural capital (the physical environment) can be complemented by a focus on our human natural capital (our young citizens). In their book *The Abundant Society,* John McKnight and Peter Block note that our roles as citizens have been subordinated to our roles as clients and consumers (McKnight and Block 2010). Many of us have become too impotent to be called real citizens and too disconnected to be effective members of a community.

Still, there is a growing recognition that we have lost a shared national purpose. We want to improve our own lives and our nation. We find agreement about integrity, fairness, altruism, responsibility, respect, and valor in all our ethnic subcultures. It is time for our governments and the marketplace to create new forms of collaboration that enhance human natural capital. Over 1200 companies have signed the 10 principles of Global Corporate Citizenship of the Global Compact launched by the United Nations in 2000 (UN n.d.). The compact covers human rights, workplace safety, justice, anti-corruption measures, and environmental sustainability.

Democracy is more than a system of government. It enables people to act together in the pursuit of common goals and aspirations. In her book *Collective Visioning: How Groups Can Work Together for a Just and Sustainable Future*, community organizer Linda Stout describes how people can rally others to work toward common goals (NAPCVI n.d.). Democracy depends upon its human ecosystem: civil alliances, social norms, and deliberative practices with a self-organizing rather than an institutional quality. Founder of Gundersen National Child Protection Training Center Victor Vieth outlined a plan to eliminate child abuse and strengthen parenthood (Vieth 2006).

Improving public policy is not always a matter of making it more responsive to the public will. It also means addressing social and political inequalities. When conflicts and disagreements arise, deliberation allows groups to arrive at a collective assessment that is more than the sum of individual opinions and preferences. The electronic social media allow us to come together more easily to create and sustain community and political movements. The health of a community, state, or nation can be measured by its social capital—its informal networks of reciprocity, trust, and mutual assistance.

The social networking organization Zocalo Public Square joined with Arizona State University and the New America Foundation to launch the nonpartisan Center for Social Cohesion (Stout 2011). The Center studies the forces that shape our sense of social unity. Its mission is to bring people together to understand our challenges today, so we can more realistically address them tomorrow.

15.9 Shift from an Individual to a Family Focus

The natural tendency is to think of persons as individuals. This is appropriate under many circumstances but not when issues affect the lives of these individuals. Mothers and fathers of minors have children and youth who depend upon them. Children and youth likewise have parents who are affected by their actions. Even a focus on children and families implies that children are freestanding individuals apart from their families. This is why "child-saver" organizations have failed. They need to be family-focused organizations in order to fulfill their missions.

As an example of an effort to shift from an individual to a family focus and provide a forum for Collaborative Systems of Care at the state level in Wisconsin, Wisconsin Cares, Inc., has proposed a Family Policy Integration Board to coordinate nine government agencies that impact families (Wisconsin Cares 2016). This board would relate to a collaborative structure in each county, tribe, or service area with an operational agreement created by an executive committee of public and private stakeholders. Such structures now exist in over 55 counties and tribes in Wisconsin.

The existing state Child Abuse and Neglect Prevention Board would be transformed into a Family Policy Integration Board that would relate to local collaboratives, facilitate collaboration and integration between agencies, evaluate the impact of legislation on families, and recommend legislative initiatives. The Board would avoid creating additional costs by drawing upon and realigning personnel from existing agencies. It would view policies from the standpoint of families rather than children and families. This means that children would not be considered freestanding individuals who are not parts of families. When a parent is not willing or able to fulfill the best interests of a child, the focus would be on helping the parent do so or on replacing the parent with a competent adoptive parent rather than placing the child in indefinite foster care without such a plan. The principle is that a child is incomplete without a competent parent.

15.10 Innovative Schools

The Knowledge Is Power Program (KIPP) is a network of charter schools that serve over 26,000 students (KIPP foundation n.d.). It offers a rigorous college-preparatory curriculum to students who would otherwise be relegated to substandard neighborhood schools. Staff visit families, so parents can sign and fulfill contracts in which they promise to help with homework, read to their kids nightly, and volunteer at school. Learning is a collaborative family-school process.

Since 1907 when Maria Montessori launched her first school in Rome, her enduring philosophy has revolved around a simple principle: curiosity drives kids to learn. Today an estimated 4000 Montessori schools operate in the United States. Clark Montessori Junior and Senior High School in Cincinnati, Ohio, is the first public junior high and high school to encourage children to follow their interests in problem-solving (Clark Montessori 2018). Collaboration is key. Each year the 600 or so students sign a contract pledging to help build the school community as well as the community outside school. Students are required to perform 200 h of community service in order to graduate.

Imagine what it would be like if each person attaining the age of legal majority pledged to abide by our nation's cultural values embedded in our laws as is required of naturalized citizens. Skeptics would say it would make no difference, but it would make a greater impression on youth than the occasional pledge of allegiance to our flag.

15.11 A National Parent Organization

The American Association of Retired Persons (AARP) is a powerful organization that lobbies for the interests of older persons (AARP n.d.). Scores of advocacy organizations for children have more or less influence over specific public policies that affect children and youth. Strikingly, there is no National Association of Parents devoted to advocate the needs of families. Parents apparently are too busy raising their children to establish and maintain a national organization.

Parents are represented now by organizations that focus on education and special needs. The National Parent Teacher Association (PTA) is the most influential (National PTA n.d.). Its agenda advocates family engagement in schools and overall improvements in general, special, and early childhood education. The PTA also is a strong advocate for increased education funding. It prioritizes the health and well-being of children through implementation of, and improvements in, nutrition laws. It aims to protect the rights of children and youth in the justice system.

The National Association of Parents with Children in Special Education (NAPCSE) renders support and assistance to parents whose children receive special education services inside and outside school (NAPCSE n.d.). It was founded to provide parents with children with special needs a sense of community and a national forum for their ideas.

The National Association for Parents of Children with Visual Impairments (NAPCVI) enables parents through the Lighthouse Guild to find information and resources for children who are blind or visually impaired (NAPCVI n.d.). The National Autism Association (NAA) responds to the most urgent needs of the autism community, providing help and hope so that everyone can reach their full potential (National Autism Organization n.d.).

The American Grandparents Association (AGA) provides networking, support, and education to caregivers (American Grandparents Association n.d.). Generations United (GU) is a national coalition dedicated to intergenerational policy programs and issues (GU n.d.). The Foundation for Grandparenting (FG) is a nonprofit organization that raises grandparent consciousness (FG n.d.). It also promotes the importance of grandparenting as a role and function that creates meaning and empowerment in later life while benefiting all family members.

These organizations perform important functions for specific interest groups, but we need an umbrella National Association of Parents (NAP) dedicated to promoting parenthood and family resources for all parents.

15.12 A Vision for the Future

The prosperity of our nation depends upon all of our children and adolescents becoming productive citizens. Our Declaration of Independence declares that all newborn babies—as our posterity—are entitled to an opportunity to become productive citizens. All adolescents deserve to work through the joys and discomforts of adolescence without having their growing bodies, minds, and personalities burdened by pregnancy and parenthood. All parents deserve to raise their adolescents without the responsibility of rearing another generation.

There is a difference between being a parent and embracing parenthood as a career. We cannot expect dependent persons to avoid parenthood until society affirms that parenthood is a rewarding, lifelong, sacrificial career for those who are capable of assuming its responsibilities. We betray their trust when we do not protect pregnant adolescents prior to childbirth from decisions that profoundly alter the courses of their lives.

Our society does not have a way of ensuring that genetic parents are competent and accountable. Legal and physical custody of a newborn is given to anyone who conceived that child regardless of that person's ability to raise a child. We do not intervene until that child has been damaged by abuse or neglect.

Most thoughtful Americans value the responsibility, integrity, opportunity, and privacy embodied in competent parenthood. When all children have competent parents with adequate resources for achieving skills and generating hope for the future, our society will have overcome juvenile ageism. This vision is not pie-in-the-sky thinking. We can move forward strongly if we act upon the simple fact that minor and dependent adult parents require legal and physical custodians themselves and therefore cannot be the custodians of other persons. They are incapable of being competent parents. This will help break the cycle of intergenerational poverty.

This vision can be achieved if we value parenthood as a vital career that requires basic managerial skills and essential resources. The Parenthood Affirmation as a part of the Birth Certificate would make explicit our implicit Parent-Society Contract. This Affirmation could only be made by those who are not under the custody or guardianship of others. This Affirmation would have a profound effect on our society by demonstrating through small but crucial actions that newborn babies are valued by our society and are full-fledged citizens with the right to have competent parents who can give them an opportunity to succeed in life.

Because our society does not articulate its expectations for parents, child neglect and abuse in the United States have reached epidemic proportions and exceed rates in all other developed nations. We only intervene after children have been damaged by neglect and abuse, often ineffectively. Enormous public expenditures on treatment, rehabilitation, and incarceration follow. This would change dramatically if our vision for America was that all of our children would be raised by competent parents.

References

AARP. https://www.aarp.org/. Accessed 6 July 2018.

American Grandparents Association. https://aga.grandparents.com/. Accessed 6 July 2018.

Boehm, C. (2012). *Moral origins: The evolution of virtue, altruism, and shame.* New York: Basic Books.

Cain, S. (2012). *Quiet: The power of introverts in a world that can't stop talking.* New York: Crown Publishing Group/Random House.

Children of the Code. (2018). Imagine growing up ashamed of your mind. http://childrenofthecode.org/. Accessed 6 July 2018.

Clark Montessori High School, Cincinnati, Ohio. (2018). https://clark.cps-k12.org/. Accessed 6 July 2018.

Foundation for Grandparenting. http://www.grandmagazine.com/. Accessed 6 July 2018.

GU [Generations United]. http://www.gu.org/. Accessed 6 July 2018.

Henderson, H. (1996). *Building a win-win world.* New York: Berrett-Koehler Publishers.

KIPP Foundation. (n.d.). Great education transforms lives. http://www.kipp.org/. Accessed 6 July 2018.

Lifton, R. J. (1989). *Thought reform and the psychology of totalism: A study of "Brainwashing" in China.* Durham: UNC Press.

McKnight, J., & Block, P. (2010). *The abundant community: Awakening the power of families and neighborhoods.* New York: Berrett-Koehler Publishers.

McNamara, R. S., & Van De Mark, B. (1996). *In retrospect: The tragedy and lessons of Vietnam.* New York: Vintage Press.

NAPCSE [National Association of Parents with Children in Special Education]. http://www.napcse.org/. Accessed 6 July 2018.

NAPCVI [National Association for Parents of Children with Visual Impairments]. *Lighthouse guild.* http://www.napvi.org/. Accessed 6 July 2018.

National Autism Association. http://nationalautismassociation.org/. Accessed 6 July 2018.

National PTA. https://www.pta.org/. Accessed 6 July 2018.

Price, M. (2010). From scorn to envy. *APA Monitor, 41*(9), 36. http://www.apa.org/monitor/2010/10/compassion.aspx. Accessed 6 July 2018.

Putnam, R. D. (2001). *Bowling alone: The collapse and revival of American community*. New York: Simon & Schuster.

Soros, G. (2011). My philanthropy. Reprinted from The *New York Review of Books*, June 22, 2011. https://www.georgesoros.com/2011/06/22/my_philanthropy/. Accessed 6 July 2018.

Stout, L. (2011). *Collective visioning: How groups can work together for a just and sustainable future*. New York: Berrett-Koehler Publishers.

United Nations. (n.d.). United Nations global compact. http://www.csrwire.com/members/12044-united-nations-global-compact. Accessed 6 July 2018.

Vieth, V. I. (2006). Unto the third generation: A call to end child abuse in the United States within 120 years (revised and expanded). *Hamline Journal of Public Law & Policy, 28*, 1.

Wisconsin Cares, Inc. (2016). Protecting our most precious asset: Our youngest citizens. A place to start: The affirmation of parenthood. http://www.wisconsincares.net/wp-content/uploads/2016/03/Parenthood_Affirmation_Proposal_11-15.pdf. Accessed 6 July 2018.

Appendix 1

Public Expenditures Related to Struggling Families (Largely Federal Funds Passed Through States to Localities)

Wisconsin executive budget 2012		
Costs of struggling families calculated by departments		
Department of Corrections		1.2 billion
Department of Health Services	8.8 billion	2.8 billion
(Medicaid—28% low income and 20% elderly 2.8 billion)		
Department of Children and Families	1.3 billion	
Department of Public Instruction	0.2 billion	
(Special education 0.54 billion (behavioral categories 0.2 billion)		
Department of Workforce Development	1.1 billion	1.2 billion
(Workforce development 0.3 billion)		
(Economic support 0.9 billion)		
Youth Aids		0.1 billion
Office of Justice Assistance		0.2 billion
	Total	7.0 billion
		(23% of $30 billion)
Wisconsin county budgets (Wisconsin Taxpayers Alliance)		
Total expenditures (2010) $5.3 billion		
Law enforcement	0.76 billion	
Jail costs	0.48 billion	
Juvenile and domestic violence	0.28 billion	
Health and human services ($2.1 billion)		
Mental health and public health (50%)	0.4 billion	
Human services	1.2 billion	
	Total	$2.36 billion
		(45% of $5.3 billion)

© Springer Nature Switzerland AG 2019
J. C. Westman, *Dealing with Child Abuse and Neglect as Public Health Problems*, https://doi.org/10.1007/978-3-030-05897-5

Appendix 2

Financial Cost of a Habitual Criminal from a Single-Parent Family Receiving Public Benefits

1. Lived at home with single mother (from birth to 13 years)	Dollar cost
TANF payments	$61,400
Social services ($2633×13)	40,200
2. Lived at home with parent (ages 13–15 years)	
Arrests by police (3)	750
Court costs (2)	5520
Detained overnight (1)	128
Probation services	6320
3. Juvenile correctional institution (ages 15 years to 15 years, 30 months)	
Arrest by police (1)	260
Court cost (1)	2770
Detained overnight (1)	128
Correctional facilities	12,690
4. Lived at home with parent (ages 15 years, 3 months to 17 years, 3 months)	
Probation (1 year)	3160
Arrest by police (1)	260
Court cost (1)	2775
5. Adult prison (ages 18–60 years; 42 years in prison)	
Court costs (3×$2775)	8320
Arrests by police (3×$260)	780
Jail detention ($128×60)	7680
Adult prison ($25,500×40)	1,071,000
Total juvenile cost	$136,361
Total adult cost	$1,087,780
Total direct cost for services	$1,224,141
Total direct cost to government	$1,350,141
Total loss of federal income taxes ($30,000 single person; $3000×42)	$126,000
Loss to national economy ($36,000×42 years)	$1,512,000
Total monetary cost to society for individual	**$2,862,141**

© Springer Nature Switzerland AG 2019
J. C. Westman, *Dealing with Child Abuse and Neglect as Public Health Problems*, https://doi.org/10.1007/978-3-030-05897-5

Index

© Springer Nature Switzerland AG 2019
J. C. Westman, *Dealing with Child Abuse and Neglect as Public Health
Problems*, https://doi.org/10.1007/978-3-030-05897-5

C

CAPTA Reauthorization Act of 2010, 27
Caregivers, 33, 34, 53
Casualties, 66
Catholic Church
  Child Dignity in the Digital World, 35
  Dominican Republic, 35
  frightening digital world, 35
  International Politics and Law Regarding
    Child Sexual Abuse, 35
Center for the Improvement of Child Caring
  (CICC), 150
Centers for Disease Control and Prevention
  (CDC), 17–19, 29
Certification process, 170, 171
Child abuse and neglect, 186
  biological processes, 28
  child fatality, 29
  child maltreatment report, 28
  child protective services, 28
  federal law, 27
  physical and mental health damage, 28
  types of maltreatment, 27
  universal prejudices, 28
  violent society, 30
Child Abuse and Neglect Prevention Board,
  183
The Child Abuse Prevention and Treatment
  Act (CAPTA), 27, 145
Child advocacy centers, 34
Childbirth, 159
Childcare systems, 55
Child Dignity in the Digital World, 35
Child exploitation, 72, 73
The Child Free-Network, 42
Childhood adversity, 173
Child in Need of Protective Services, 3, 86
Childism, 46
Child maltreatment, 27, 70, 72
Child Online Protection Act, 57
Child-parent relationship
  children as citizens, 124
  children as family members, 123, 124
  children as private property, 123
Child/parent unit, 61, 66
Child pornography, 35, 36
Child protective services (CPS), 28
Childrearing, 83–88, 90, 92, 94, 97
Children as adults
  adolescent childbearing, 61–63
  adolescent childbirth, 61
  adolescent pregnancy, 61–63, 65
  adult responsibilities, 59, 60

child-parent unit, 61
freestanding persons, 61, 62
punitive adult policies, 60
testify in court, 60
Children's Bureau report Child Maltreatment
  2015, 29
Children's Defense Fund, 1, 159
Children's rights
  American Civil War, 107
  attachment bonding
    affiliative, 114
    archeologists and anthropologists
     building, 112
    attachment styles, 116
    children's behavior, 112
    interpersonal relationships and market
     economies, 112
    lifetime health records, 112
    newborn babies, 112
    nurturing, 115
    parent-child relationship, 113
    sexual, 115
    stable family relationships, 113
    succoring bonding system, 113, 114
    working models, 113
  capacity and experience, 108
  childhood and adolescence, 107
  civil rights, 109, 110
  developing mind
    eye-to-eye contact, 116
    father relationships, 118
    learning, 117
    self-generated play, 117
    stable mental images, 116
    us/them memes, 117, 118
  developmental needs of babies, 111
  functions, 108
  habit of happiness, 107
  moral rights, minors, 108, 109
  newborn babies, 108
  right to competent parents, 111
  Save the Children, 107
Child-saver organizations, 183
Child Trends survey, 96
Child Wellbeing Study, 97
Cigarette smoking, 16
Citizens, 182, 185, 186
The Civil Rights Movement, 40
Civilized behavior, 118
Classism, 40, 41
Collaboration, 177, 179, 181–184
Collaborative systems of care (CSC), 141, 146
Collective Visioning, 182

CPSIA information can be obtained
at www.ICGtesting.com
Printed in the USA
LVHW080954270319
612007LV00001B/1/P